A Colour Atlas of

ALLERGY

William F. Jackson
MA, MB, BChir, MRCP
Medical Producer,
British Medical Television.
Formerly Honorary Consultant in Allergy
Department of Medicine
Guy's Hospital
London

Rino Cerio
BSc, MB, BS, MRCP
Senior Registrar and Tutor in Dermatology
St John's Hospital for Diseases of the Skin
London

With a chapter on Allergic Disorders of the Eye *by*

David L. Easty
MD, FRCS
Professor of Ophthalmology
University of Bristol

Wolfe Medical Publications Ltd

Copyright © William F. Jackson and Rino Cerio, 1988
Published by Wolfe Medical Publications Ltd, 1988
Printed by W.S. Cowell Ltd, Ipswich, England
ISBN 0 7234 0914 5 Cased edition
ISBN 0 7234 1600 1 Paperback edition
Paperback edition © 1989

For a full list of Wolfe Medical Atlases, plus
forthcoming titles and details of our surgical,
dental and veterinary Atlases, please write to
Wolfe Publishing Ltd, 2-16 Torrington Place,
London WC1E 7LT.

General Editor, Wolfe Medical Atlases:
G. Barry Carruthers, MD(Lond)

CONTENTS

ACKNOWLEDGEMENTS

We gratefully acknowledge the help of friends, colleagues and organisations who have helped us by allowing us to reproduce slides from their collections or in many other ways.

Mr T.R. Bull

Dr P.J Ciclatira

Mr J. Daws

Dr Martha Dynski-Klein

Dr C. Farthing

Mr M.J. Gleeson

Mrs Sue Gynes

Dr D. Geraint James and Dr P. R. Studdy

Dr L.K. Jackson

Prof M.H. Lessof

Dr D.M. MacDonald

Dr R.S. Wells

Dr L.J.F. Youlten

Guy's Hospital Medical School

Allen and Hanburys Ltd

Bencard (Beecham Group)

Clement Clarke International Ltd

Pharmacia G.B. Ltd

We also thank Barbara, Clare and Ian Jackson and Soraya Cerio for their continuing encouragement and support.

1   MECHANISMS IN ALLERGY

The body's immune system is divided functionally into *innate* (non-specific) and *adaptive* (specific) components.

THE INNATE IMMUNE SYSTEM
First line defence of the body against infection is provided by the innate immune system, which consists of a range of physical, chemical and cellular mechanisms. These mechanisms are active in all normal individuals, and prevent most potential infections by pathogens. But they are not specific, and they are not enhanced by repeated infection.

THE ADAPTIVE IMMUNE SYSTEM
The adaptive immune system comes into play when the innate immune system has failed to deal with a foreign antibody. The adaptive system involves both cellular and humoral mechanisms and is characterised by specific immunological memory, so that repeat exposure to the organism or antigen at a later date provokes an enhanced immune response. This enhanced response pro-

Table 1. The innate immune system

Biochemical defences
Lysozyme in mucosal secretions
Complement
Acute phase proteins—e.g. Interferon and C-reactive protein (CRP)
Sebaceous gland secretions
Commensal gut and vaginal organisms
Spermine in semen
Acid in stomach

Physical defences
Skin
Cilia in respiratory tract
Mucus

Cellular defences
Phagocytes
Natural killer (NK) cells

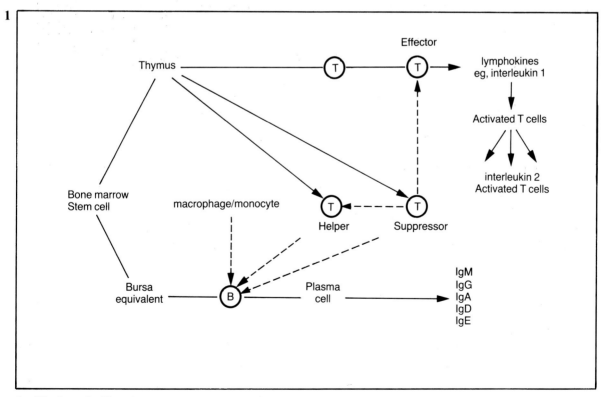

1   The lymphoid system

duces a life-long immunity to diseases such as diphtheria and measles following first infection and can be said to be 'appropriate' in these circumstances. Clinical allergy is concerned mainly with the effects of apparently *inappropriate* function of the adaptive immune system (though abnormalities of the innate immune system are sometimes also of significance).

Adaptive immunity is mediated by the lymphoid system (1). This system can respond to a variety of antigenic foreign material, irrespective of whether the material is potentially harmful or not. It produces two major populations of immunocompetent cells—thymus dependent or T cells and bursa dependent or B cells. These effect, respectively, cell-mediated and antibody-mediated specific immunity.

The humoral immune response
Antibodies are produced by B cells in response to an antigenic stimulus, but this process requires the involvement of macrophages and helper T cells. T cell populations modulate both the cellular and humoral immune responses through a complex set of sub-populations of suppressor, helper and activated T lymphocytes. The products of the B cells, antibodies, are found in five classes: IgM, IgG, IgA, IgD and IgE. Each has a unique structure and function.

The cellular immune response
The products of the cellular immune response, antigen sensitised lymphocytes, are composed of several sub-populations of T cells, with varying physicochemical, antigenic and functional characteristics. Upon encountering antigens, the immune system may variably activate a number of effector systems, including the mediators from basophil granules, complement, prostaglandins, kinins and lymphokines. These stimulate the body's specific and non-specific defence mechanisms of inflammation. At the same time, the response creates a reserve of 'memory cells' for future demands.

ABNORMALITIES OF THE IMMUNE RESPONSE
A failure of any part of the immune system may predispose to infection, malignancy or allergy. A depressed immune response is not always easy to diagnose clinically, and may be secondary to a number of causes (see Chapter 10).

Apparently immune responses are not always triggered by sensitization to antigens. So called 'pseudo-allergic' reactions may occur in response to various drugs, for example, and these may cause anaphylaxis, haemolytic anaemia, immune complex disease and delayed cell-mediated responses in non-sensitized individuals. The mechanisms involve direct effects on prostaglandin release, mast cell or complement activity.

In addition, non-specific tissue mechanisms of inflammation can be triggered by immune reactions which become amplified to produce clinical features identical to immunologically mediated diseases. The bronchial response to histamine, for example, may often be a combined effect of tissue reactivity and allergy in asthmatics. In the gut, IgE release provoked by infective agents or foods may produce a series of physiological consequences including blood vessel dilatation, oedematous villi, local cellular infiltration and leakage of plasma proteins into the intestinal lumen. Again, a minor immunological response can provoke major pathophysiological consequences.

Table 2. Comparison of human immunoglobulin classes

Immunoglobin class	Serum concentration (adult)	Molecular weight	Light chain	Heavy chain
IgG	9.5-16.5 g/L	160,000	K & L	ყ
IgA	0.9-4.5 g/L	170,000 and polymer	K & L	α
IgM	0.6-2.0 g/L	960,000	K & L	π
IgD	3.0-400 mg/L	184,000	K & L	δ
IgE	10.0-130 mg/L	188,000	K & L	ε

There are four sub-classes of IgG. These reflect four distinct types of heavy chain. Normal percentage totals of the sub-classes of IgG are as follows: IgG_1 65%; IgG_2 23%; IgG_3 8%; IgG_4 4%.

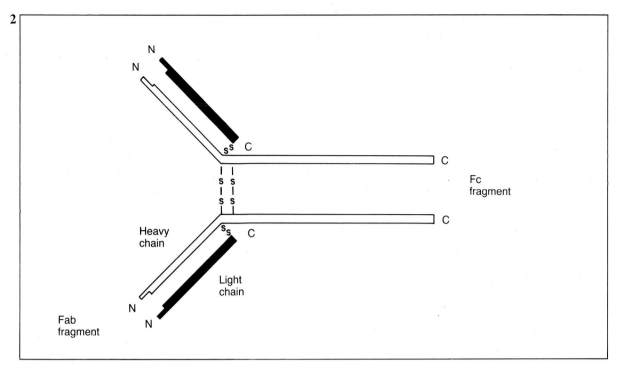

2 The basic structure of immunoglobulins. Each immunoglobin molecule consists of two identical light polypeptide chains and two heavy polypeptide chains, linked together by disulphide bonds. Note the position of the amino (N) and carboxyl (C) terminal ends of the peptide chains. The amino terminal ends are the antigen binding sites, hence this end of the molecule is known as the Fab fragment. The Fc fragment has sites for complement fixation, reactivity with rheumatoid factors, membrane transmission, macrophage fixation and regulation of catabolism.

Table 3. Biological properties of major human immunoglobulin classes

Immuno-globulin	Half life (days)	Role	Characteristic properties			
			Complement fixation	Crosses placenta	Fixes to mast/ basophil cells	Cytophilic binding to macrophages
IgG	18-23	Precipitins, antitoxins	+	+	−	+
IgA	5-6.5	Surface protection	−	−	−	−
IgM	5	Agglutinins, opsonins, lysins, earliest antibody	−	−	−	−
IgD	2-8	On lymphocyte surface of newborn	?	−	−	−
IgE	2.3	Involved in atopy. Raised in parasitic infections	−	+	−	−

Hypersensitivity reactions

Deleterious or inappropriate immune responses are termed hypersensitivity reactions. The Gell and Coombs classification divides these reactions into four types according to their immunopathological mechanisms, but in many, if not most, clinical situations more than one immunological mechanism may be involved, though one reaction type may predominate. In allergic asthma, for example, the early reaction to an allergen is mediated by IgE, but later phases run a more prolonged time course and may involve immune complexes or cellular infiltration.

Classification of hypersensitivity reactions

Type I

This type of response is triggered by antigen which has penetrated body surfaces, e.g. skin, respiratory or gastrointestinal tract. The antigen combines with cell bound (reaginic) antibody on mast or basophil cell membranes. Bridging of IgE molecules on the mast cell surface triggers an immediate local release of vasoactive amines, initiated by a fall in cellular cyclic AMP. This response is normally transient and limited by the influence of suppressor T cells. When IgE antibody reaches higher levels this response can lead to urticaria or asthma, due to the release of histamine and other mediators. In the extreme case this mediator release can lead to acute anaphylaxis, which is potentially fatal (e.g. following penicillin injection or an insect sting in a sensitized patient).

Atopic patients have a familial tendency to develop abnormal hypersensitivity to common allergens. The atopic trait may be defined as the spontaneous tendency of an individual to produce high levels of IgE antibodies against one or more common antigens, in association with antigen-provoked disorders in which reaginic mechanisms can be identified. Examples include extrinsic allergic asthma, allergic rhinitis, allergic conjunctivitis, urticaria and atopic eczema.

Type II

This response is initiated by antibody reacting with antigenic components of cell or tissue elements. Complement fixation or K cell lysis lead to damage. The classic example is the reaction following an incompatible blood transfusion. Some drugs can adsorb to cell membranes and immunologically cause haemolysis, agranulocytosis or thrombocytopenia. A similar clinical effect may be produced by low concentrations of lymphocytotoxins, as in systemic lupus erythematosus (SLE). Antireceptor antibody can also have a blocking effect, as in myasthenia gravis.

Type III

This response occurs when antigen reacts in the tissue spaces with potentially precipitating antibody, forming microprecipitates in and around small blood vessels and causing secondary damage to cells. When antigen is in excess, soluble circulating immune complexes are formed and deposited in the endothelial lining of blood vessel walls or the basement membrane, fixing complement and causing local inflammation. This inflammation may be acute, as in serum sickness, with fever, vasculitis, skin rash, proteinuria and joint inflammation; or it may be chronic, as in SLE, uveitis, vasculitis or glomerulonephritis.

Type IV

Several different types of immune reaction can produce delayed hypersensitivity. Unlike other types of hypersensitivity, they cannot be transferred from one individual to another by serum, but can be transferred by certain T lymphocytes. The type IV reaction involves active sensitized T lymphocytes, which respond specifically to allergen by the release of lymphokines and/or the development of cytotoxicity. Locally the type IV reaction is manifested by the infiltration of cells at the site of antigen injection. Lymphokines are responsible for the recruitment of lymphocytes and the activation of local macrophages. Cells are identified as targets for cell-mediated immune attack by surface antigenic determinants which are immunogenic in the host. These may be histocompatibility antigens, new membrane antigens induced by viral, bacterial or other infection, tumour-specific antigens or native surface antigens involved in autoimmune reactions.

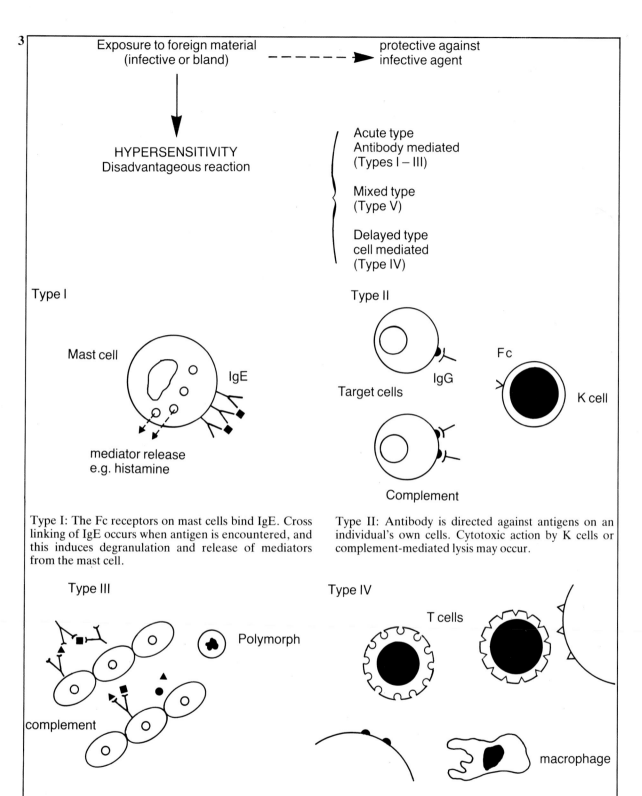

3

Exposure to foreign material
(infective or bland)

- - - - - - → protective against
infective agent

HYPERSENSITIVITY
Disadvantageous reaction

Acute type
Antibody mediated
(Types I – III)

Mixed type
(Type V)

Delayed type
cell mediated
(Type IV)

Type I

Mast cell

IgE

mediator release
e.g. histamine

Type I: The Fc receptors on mast cells bind IgE. Cross linking of IgE occurs when antigen is encountered, and this induces degranulation and release of mediators from the mast cell.

Type II

Target cells

IgG

Fc

K cell

Complement

Type II: Antibody is directed against antigens on an individual's own cells. Cytotoxic action by K cells or complement-mediated lysis may occur.

Type III

Polymorph

complement

Type III: Immune complexes are deposited in tissues. Local damage occurs due to complement activation and attraction of polymorphs to the site of deposition.

Type IV

T cells

macrophage

Type IV: Antigen-sensitized T cells release lymphokines following a secondary contact with the same antigen. Lymphokines induce inflammatory reactions and activate macrophages, which release mediators.

Key

▲ ■ ● Antigens
Antibodies
Membrane receptors

3 Classification of hypersensitivity reactions

Table 4. Human immune complex diseases

Type	Allergen	Disease
Infection	Bacteria	Subacute bacterial endocarditis
		Meningococcal infection
		Leprosy
	Protozoal	Malaria
	Viral	Hepatitis B
Neoplasia	Tumour antigen	Lymphoma
		Carcinoma
Autoimmunity	IgG	Rheumatoid arthritis
	Nucleic acids	Systemic lupus erythematosus
Exogenous	Drugs, e.g. penicillin, hydrallazine	Serum sickness Systemic lupus erythematosus syndrome
	Occupational allergens, e.g. farmers' lung (Micropolyspora faeni)	Extrinsic allergic alveolitis
	Dietary, e.g. gluten sensitivity	Coeliac disease
		Dermatitis herpetiformis

2 INVESTIGATION OF ALLERGIC DISORDERS

The patient's history is of particular importance in reaching a diagnosis of allergic disorder. In hay fever, for example, the diagnosis is usually evident from a combination of the nature of the symptoms, their timing, and their association with pollen in the air.

Examination of the patient may show relevant abnormalities—for example, eczema, urticaria, rhinitis or signs of asthma; or it may show a clearly non-allergic cause for the symptoms.

Further investigations are often helpful in the confirmation of suspected allergic reactions or in the unravelling of previously unsuspected allergy, but the common clinical allergies are usually investigated by a fairly small range of tests. Many more complex tests of immune function are available, but these are mainly used for research purposes and in immunodeficiency states (see Chapter 10) and autoimmune diseases (see Chapter 9).

4 Self-adminstered allergy questionnaire, (as used at Guy's Hospital, London) can help both doctor and patient to make best use of subsequent consulatation time (see following pages).

Note that the questionnaire asks about:
the symptoms
their timing
provoking factors
previous treatment
relevant social history
family history
early childhood
possible provocation by foods.

Significant responses can be followed up in the consultation. A simple symptom chart, kept by the patient for a few days or weeks may also be helpful in the search for provoking and relieving factors.

4

ALLERGY CLINIC Patient's Questionnaire

While you are waiting for your allergy tests and for the doctor to see you, you can help us by filling in as many parts of this form as you can.

Date_____ Surname_____
Present Occupation_____ First Names_____
Past Occupation_____ Address_____
Hospital_____ Hosp. No._____ Date of Birth_____
Height_____ Weight_____ Place of Birth_____
If you have lived abroad, when did you move (back) to England?_____

Please underline any of the following symptoms which you have had, and say when they started.
                                           Year of onset
Asthma, Wheezing, Tightness   _____
Attacks of Bronchitis or Cough   _____
Persistent Shortness of Breath   _____
Irritation of Eyes or Swelling of Eyelids _____
Irritation of Throat and Mouth   _____
Runny Nose, Sneezing, Blocked Nose, Sinusitis _____
Eczema or Skin Irritation, Nettle Rash or Other Rash _____
Diarrhoea, Vomiting, Constipation, Bloated Feeling, Wind or Indigestion _____
Migraine or Recurrent Headache _____
Sleep Disturbance _____
Any Other _____

Have you noticed that symptoms come on:
1 At any special time of the day or night Yes/No. If Yes, when?_____
2 At all times of the year Yes/No. If Yes, which months are worse?_____
3 Only at a particular time of the year Yes/No. If Yes, when?_____
4 In any particular room of the house Yes/No. If Yes, which one?_____
5 At work Yes/No. If Yes, are there materials, dusts or fumes which bring on or increase your symptoms?_____

Please underline which of the following can make your symptoms worse:
House Dust   Bed Making   Vacuuming/Dusting   Grass   Flowers   Trees
Animals – which?_____
Foods – which?_____
Aspirin?_____ Any other drugs?_____
Tobacco Smoke   Changes in Temperature   Exertion   Stress/Anxiety   Bronchitis
Others – please name_____

cont/sheet 2 . . .

14

What treatment have you had? (Please circle and add 'helpful' or 'no help').

1 Tablets of _____

2 Inhaler, e.g. Ventolin, Medihaler, Alupent _____
_____

3 Intal, Rynacrom

4 Becotide, Beconase

5 Steroid Tablets, e.g. Prednisolone, Cortisone or Injection, e.g. Synacthen

6 Skin treatment – Steroid Creams

7 Desensitising Injections

Accommodation

Are your symptoms better or worse since you last moved house?

Please compare:	Present House	Previous House
Age of house	_____	_____
Damp – near river	_____	_____
Damp – structural reasons	_____	_____

Holidays

When staying away from home, are your symptoms usually: Better/Worse/The Same

Animals

What animals do you have at home? _____

How long have you had them? _____

Also:

Have you ever smoked?   Yes/No

Do you smoke now?   Yes/No   If Yes, please give details _____

Have you ever attended any other hospital for your allergy? Yes/No. If Yes, give details _____
_____
_____

Do any of your family suffer from the following (if possible, state diagnosis)

	Father	Mother	Father's Relatives	Mother's Relatives	Brothers/ Sisters	Children
Allergies	_____	_____	_____	_____	_____	_____
Chest disorder	_____	_____	_____	_____	_____	_____
Skin disorder	_____	_____	_____	_____	_____	_____
Hay Fever	_____	_____	_____	_____	_____	_____

What previous illnesses have you had? _____
_____
_____

cont/sheet 3 . . .

Food related symptoms

1 If any foods upset you, or if they have done in the past, please state the year in which each one started to upset you and name the foods concerned.

_____
_____
_____

2 What symptoms do you (or did you) get?

_____

3 How long after taking the food? (for each symptom)

_____
_____
_____

4 If it is more than six months since you first had symptoms following food can you say what would happen if you take this food now?
Would the symptoms be: BETTER/WORSE/THE SAME/DON'T KNOW *or* would you have no symptoms?_____

5 If you still avoid this food, for how long have you done this?
a) Three months   b) 3–6 months   c) 6–12 months   d) More than a year

---

FOR CHILDREN ONLY

Was the child entirely breast fed?_____
If so, for how long?_____
Age of starting to eat: Cow's Milk_____ Milk Powder_____
Bread_____ Rusks or Cereal_____ Eggs_____

Were there difficulties with feeding?   At what age?_____
Screaming attacks?   At what age?_____
Vomiting?   At what age?_____
Diarrhoea?   At what age?_____

Were there any particular foods which brought on symptoms e.g. Wheezing, Skin Irritation, Swellings, etc._____ How long after eating this food?_____

Were there any particular foods which the child disliked?

_____

Underline any particular problems: Bed Wetting, Fidgetting, Cannot Concentrate, Aggressive, Overactive, Sleeps Badly, Depressed, Moody, Difficult. Any others_____
What previous illnesses has she/he had (please include frequent Sore Throats, Earache or Infections)_____

Does either parent smoke at home Yes/No. If Yes, details please_____

SKIN-PRICK TESTS

Skin-prick tests are usually less important than the history in the diagnosis of allergic conditions, but they often provide useful confirmatory evidence of reaction to suspected allergens. They are simple to carry out and interpret, but they do not give absolute evidence of clinically relevant allergy. A patient with asthma may, for example, show positive skin-prick reactions to allergens which do not trigger bronchospasm on direct challenge; or he may have a positive challenge test with allergens which give negative skin-prick results.

In the case of respiratory tract symptoms provoked by pollen, house dust mite excreta or animal dander there is a 75 per cent agreement between the results of provocation tests and skin tests. The concordance between skin test results and symptoms from *ingested* allergens is much lower—indeed, skin-prick testing is only of limited help in the diagnosis of food-allergic disease (see page 89).

Skin-prick tests differ from scratch tests and intracutaneous tests. Scratch testing is imprecise and unhelpful. Intracutaneous tests, in which allergens are injected more deeply into the skin, are reproducible and have an occasional role; but they are in general less specific, less well authenticated and more hazardous than prick tests.

Table 5. Allergens commonly included in skin-prick test batteries in the UK*

Pollens:	Grass (mixed) Trees (e.g. silver birch and plane)
House dust mite	
Domestic animals:	Cat Dog Horse
Moulds:	*Alternaria* *Cladosporium* *Aspergillus*
Foods:	Milk Egg
Controls:	Saline - negative Histamine - positive

*Many additional and more specific extracts are available for use in selected patients, and the standard battery of allergens varies from one centre to another and between countries—depending upon the locally prevalent allergens.

5

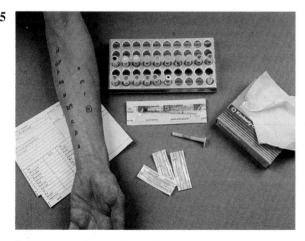

6

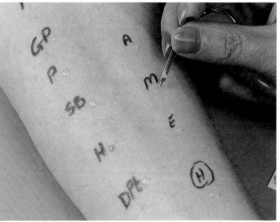

5 Equipment for skin-prick testing includes alcohol swabs or tissues for skin preparation, a skin marker pen, appropriate allergen extracts with control solutions of saline and histamine, and skin lances (some operators prefer to use 25G needles). Skin lances which have been pre-coated with freeze-dried allergens are also now available. A measuring rule and a report form are also required.

Because of the slight risk of an anaphylactic reaction, it is essential that a medically qualified person is immediately available, together with injectable 1 in 1000 adrenaline (epinephrine) solution, antihistamines and other resuscitation facilities.

6 Skin-prick testing. The skin is cleaned, prick sites are marked and a small drop of each allergen solution is placed on the skin. A lance is introduced through the drop to a depth of about 1 mm into the skin, and pulled out, raising the skin in the process. The skin should not bleed. The site is blotted dry. The lance can be wiped thoroughly dry with a sterile swab and re-used with another solution in the same patient—but never in another patient.

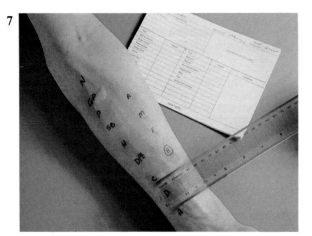

7

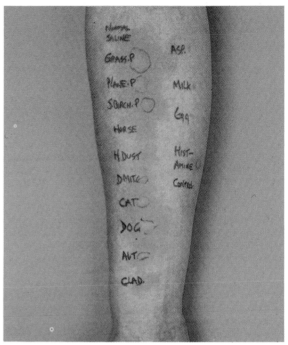

8

7 Reading the prick test result. The maximum reaction is usually seen after 15-20 minutes. The saline control should be negative (unless the patient has dermographism—see **55**). The histamine control should be positive—recent antihistamine administration may cause a negative result, and this will invalidate other negative reactions. Positive results are best recorded by measuring the size of the weal in millimetres—the flare should be ignored. There is a reasonable correlation between the size of the weal and the significance of different inhaled allergens in a single patient. An immediate response is good evidence for a type I allergic reaction.

Later reactions may occur as well as or instead of the immediate response. Sometimes a more ill-defined response—usually a soft swelling—may occur at the site from 8 to 24 hours after the test. This probably represents immune-complex deposition in a type III reaction, but its clinical significance is often unclear. It may sometimes be correlated with symptoms of delayed onset after allergen exposure or with a biphasic response to bronchial challenge testing (see **166**).

A late reaction developing after 24-48 hours is uncommon after testing with the usual prick test allergens and is likely to represent delayed (type IV) hypersensitivity. Its relevance to the common allergic diseases is unclear, but type IV responses of this kind to a battery of micro-organism antigens are an important test of cell-mediated immune function. They are used in the assessment of immunodeficiency (see Chapter 10).

8 A multiple positive prick test result. This patient had symptoms of hay fever from April to August, which correlates with the positive reactions to grass, plane and silver birch pollens. He also developed nasal and eye symptoms on contact with cats—but, despite the positive skin test, dogs did not cause his symptoms, and there was nothing to suggest that *Alternaria* contributed to his rhinitis. Note that the other allergens gave negative results—the flare reactions should be regarded as a non-specific reaction, as there was no measurable weal.

PATCH TESTS

Patch tests are used principally to identify causative allergens in suspected allergic contact dermatitis. They should not be used in patients with acute eczema as results here are misleading.

The allergens are formulated in appropriate concentrations and placed in shallow aluminium wells of about 1 cm^2—Finn chambers. The wells are applied in strips to the patient's back and kept in place by hypo-allergenic tape. The skin is marked appropriately, and the patient asked to keep the area dry.

The patches are removed after 48 hours and the skin examined for a positive response, characterized by itching and erythematous swelling, often accompanied by vesiculation, all of which may extend beyond the margin of the patch in strongly positive responses. This reaction represents a cell-mediated delayed hypersensitivity (type IV) response. Irritants may cause a rather similar response, but the reaction is commonly painful rather than itchy, and epidermal necrosis may occur.

With most substances the allergic response is maximal at 48 hours, but some chemicals (e.g. neomycin) cause a later response, so a second reading of the patches at 96 hours is routine, and even later responses should be reported by the patient.

Patch testing is simple and clinically useful, but the results are not always easy to interpret. The concentration and presentation of the allergen is critical, and the distinction between an allergic and an irritant response is not always clear.

Standard contact allergen batteries have been developed in different areas of the world to include most of the common allergens in contact dermatitis. These include metallic ions, rubber accelerators and antioxidants, topical drugs and other sensitising substances. The composition of these batteries will vary from place to place and from time to time.

Table 6   A typical battery of patch test substances

	Substance	Concentration
1	Nickel Sulphate	5%
2	Bronopol	0.5%
3	Colophony	20%
4	Chlorocresol	2%
5	P.P.D.	0.5%
6	M.B.T.	2%
7	Formalin	1%
8	Potassium Dichromate	0.5%
9	Wool Alcohols	30%
10	Epoxy Resin (Araldite)	1%
11	Primin	0.01%
12	Neomycin	20%
13	Cobalt Chloride	1%
14	Dowicil 200	1%
15	Parabens	15%
16	Thiuram-mix	1%
17	Mercapto-mix	2%
18	Perfume-mix	8%
19	Black Rubber mix	0.6%
20	Carba-mix	3%
21	Quinoline mix	6%
22	Ethylenediamine	1%
23	P.T.B.P. Resin	1%
24	Kathon CG	100ppm
25	Benzocaine	5%
26	Balsam of Peru	25%
27	Imidazolidinyl Urea (G115)	2%

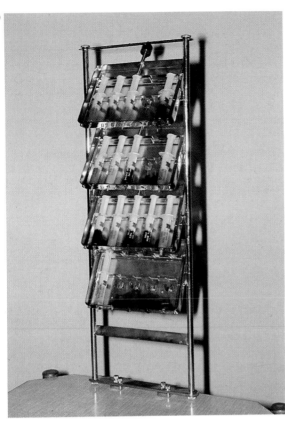

9 A battery of sensitising substances. In this case those recommended by the International Contact Dermatitis Research Group, used at standard dilutions.

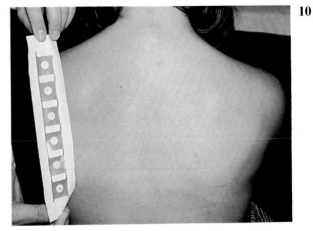

10 Aluminium wells mounted on hypo-allergenic tape and ready for application to the back.

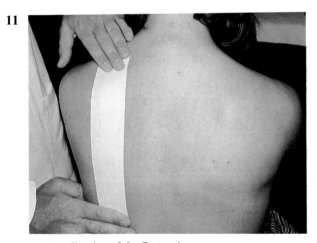

11 Application of the first strip.

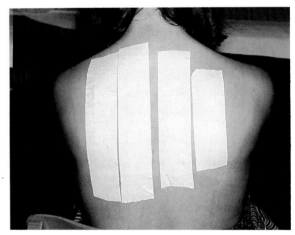

12 The complete skin test battery is now in place.

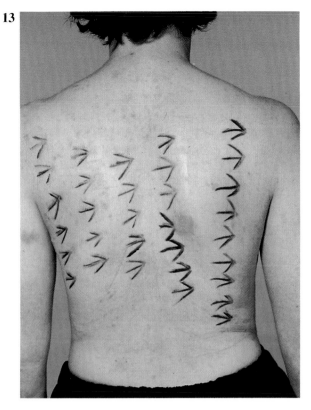

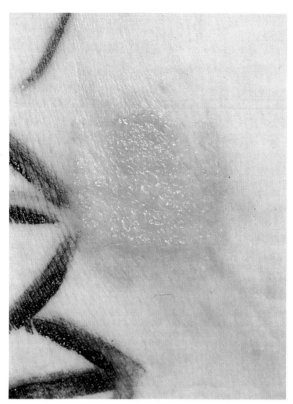

13 **Patch tests read at 48 hours**. One strongly positive result stands out.

14 **Positive patch test** from **13**, in this case to *Primula* in a 37-year-old woman (in the USA poison ivy often gives a similar reaction). Note the vesicular reaction on a base of erythema and swelling.

EOSINOPHILIA

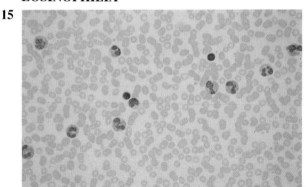

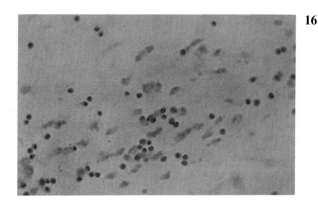

15 **Blood eosinophilia**. An eosinophil count of more than 4 per cent of total white cells may occur in atopic subjects, though massive eosinophilia is unusual and requires investigation—e.g. for intestinal parasites.

16 **Sputum eosinophilia**. This is common in asthma, and nasal eosinophilia is often found in nasal allergy, but neither finding is of direct help in management, and these investigations are not routine in most centres.

SERUM IMMUNOGLOBULINS

Serum immunoglobulin levels may be measured (for normal levels see page 8). This is an essential part of the investigation of immunodeficiency. In atopic individuals the IgE level is often elevated, and the IgA level is occasionally depressed, but type I allergic responses can occur with a normal serum IgE level. A consistent grossly elevated IgE level is often associated with intestinal parasitic infestation and should not be attributed to atopy alone without further investigation.

THE RADIOALLERGOSORBENT TEST (RAST)

The concentration of circulating IgE is very low (see page 8) and it is not possible to measure the level of IgE antibodies to specific antigens directly. This can be overcome by the RAST method.

In general, the RAST method produces results comparable with skin-prick testing in type 1 allergic disorders. It is an in-vitro technique and the blood sample can be collected away from the laboratory; but it does not provide immediate information and it is expensive. In addition, a theoretical objection is that IgE RASTs cannot detect possible IgG mediated reactions, which may conceivably be detected on skin testing. So the extent of use of the RAST method varies from one centre to another, and its role in the clinical diagnosis of allergy is not fully defined.

17

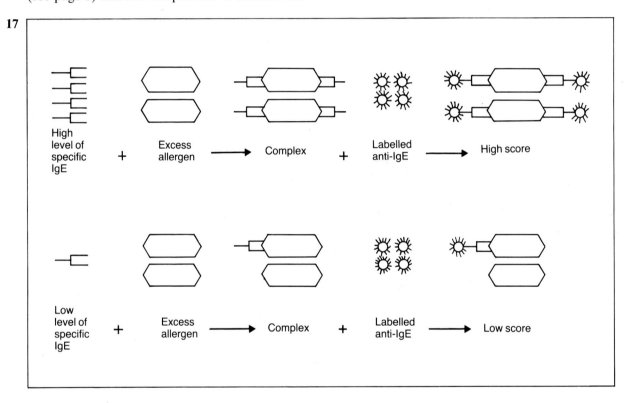

17 The RAST method. The allergen under test is bound to insoluble particles (usually on a cellulose disc), and these are incubated with the patient's serum. IgE antibodies to the antigen in the serum will bind to the sensitized particles, forming a complex. A radioactively labelled antiserum to IgE is added, the insoluble particles are separated (the disc is washed) and their radioactivity assessed. The resulting 'RAST score' varies directly in proportion with the concentration of specific IgE in the patient's serum.

OTHER INVESTIGATIONS

Challenge tests may be carried out in organs other than the skin. Thus suspected allergens may be inhaled in *bronchial* or *nasal challenge tests*, and their effects assessed by measurements of pulmonary or nasal airways resistance (see **126** and **166**). It is often difficult to distinguish allergic and irritant responses when these methods are used, but they are sometimes helpful in diagnosis and in assessing response to therapy.

Similarly, *oral challenge* with specific foods may be of help in the assessment of food allergic disease, usually following a period on a diet which excludes the allergen (see page 90 and **197**).

Radiology has a role in allergic disease of the respiratory tract (see Chapters 6 and 7) and the gut (see Chapter 8).

A number of other tests of *organic function* may, of course, be called for, depending upon the presenting clinical problem.

End-organ *biopsy* may also be of help—e.g. in many skin disorders (see Chapter 3), in gluten-sensitive enteropathy (see **192-199**) and in some autoimmune disorders (see Chapter 9).

Biopsy specimens may be examined histologically and by *immunofluorescent techniques*. In '*direct immunofluorescence*' a fluorescein-labelled reagent specific for human immunoglobulin or complement is used to reveal their deposition in the tissues—most commonly the skin (e.g. see **63**, **66** and **71**). '*Indirect immunofluorescence*' is used to reveal autoantibodies. Here, cryostat sections of tissue containing the relevant antigens are incubated with the patient's serum. A fluorescein-labelled reagent is then added, thus revealing the sites at which immunoglobulin has become bound to the tissue section.

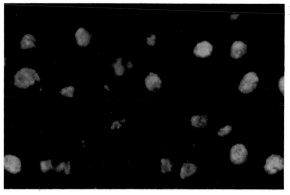

18 Antinuclear antibody as revealed by indirect immunofluorescence. The test serum came from a patient with systemic lupus erythematosus (SLE—see Chapter 9).

Table 7. Organelles and tissues to which autoantibodies which can be identified by indirect immunofluorescence

---

- Nuclei
- Mitochondria
- Smooth muscle
- Striated muscle
- Skin—basement membrane and intercellular substance
- Thyroid microsomes
- Gastric parietal cells
- Adrenal glomerulosa cells
- Pancreatic islet cells

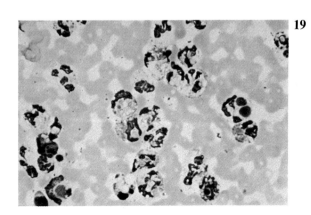

19 Lupus erythematosus cells (LE cells). These can be found in the blood of 90 per cent of patients with SLE. The LE cell is a polymorphonuclear leucocyte in which characteristic inclusions of nuclear material are found within the cytoplasm after the blood has been left standing.

Table 8. Some autoantibodies which can be identified by methods other than indirect immunofluorescence

Autoantibodies to	Method	Clinical association
DNA	1) Radioimmunoassay (RIA) 2) Enzyme linked immunosorbent assay (ELISA) 3) *Crithidia* immunofluorescence	SLE and other multisystem autoimmune disorders
RNA protein (RNP)	1) Agglutination 2) Immunodiffusion	Mixed connective tissue disease (MCD) and Raynaud's phenomenon
IgG	1) Agglutination 2) RIA 3) ELISA	Rheumatoid arthritis
Acetylcholine receptor	RIA	Myasthenia gravis
Glomerular basement membrane	RIA	Goodpasture's syndrome
Thyroglobulin	Agglutination	Hashimoto's disease
Intrinsic factor	RIA	Pernicious anaemia

INVESTIGATING THE ENVIRONMENT

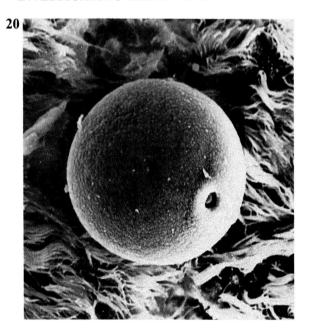

20

20 Grass pollen grain (EM × 1500). In the UK and Europe pollen from various grasses, including the crested dog's tail, fescue, foxtail, meadow rye, timothy, cocksfoot and brome is a common cause of allergic rhinitis, conjunctivitis and asthma. Tree pollens and mould spores are other causes of seasonal symptoms.

In North America, ragweed pollen is a common cause of symptoms, while other pollens are important elsewhere, e.g. mulberry pollen around the Mediterranean and prosoba tree pollens in the Middle East.

Symptoms are usually caused by airborne pollens, and an atmospheric 'pollen count' can be obtained by sampling air which is sucked through a special chamber which deposits the pollen grains onto a sticky plate. The pollen count provides a somewhat crude guide to the likely severity of symptoms in hay fever sufferers.

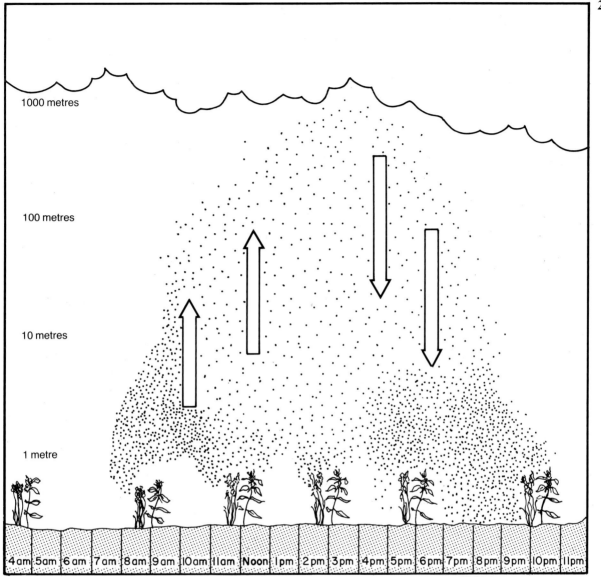

1000 metres

100 metres

10 metres

1 metre

|4am|5am|6am|7am|8am|9am|10am|11am|Noon|1pm|2pm|3pm|4pm|5pm|6pm|7pm|8pm|9pm|10pm|11pm|

21 The weather affects the pollen count. Pollen is only released in large quantities on warm and sunny days. For grasses in the UK the peak of the 'pollen season' occurs during June and July. Pollen is released in the morning, but as the air heats up it is carried high into the air during the middle of the day, descending again as the air cools in the late afternoon. The highest pollen counts therefore usually occur in mid-morning and late afternoon. Cities stay hotter for longer, so the pollen count often stays high well into the evening, whereas it falls earlier in rural areas. Heavy rain usually results in a dramatic fall in the pollen count.

pollen grains
per cubic metre

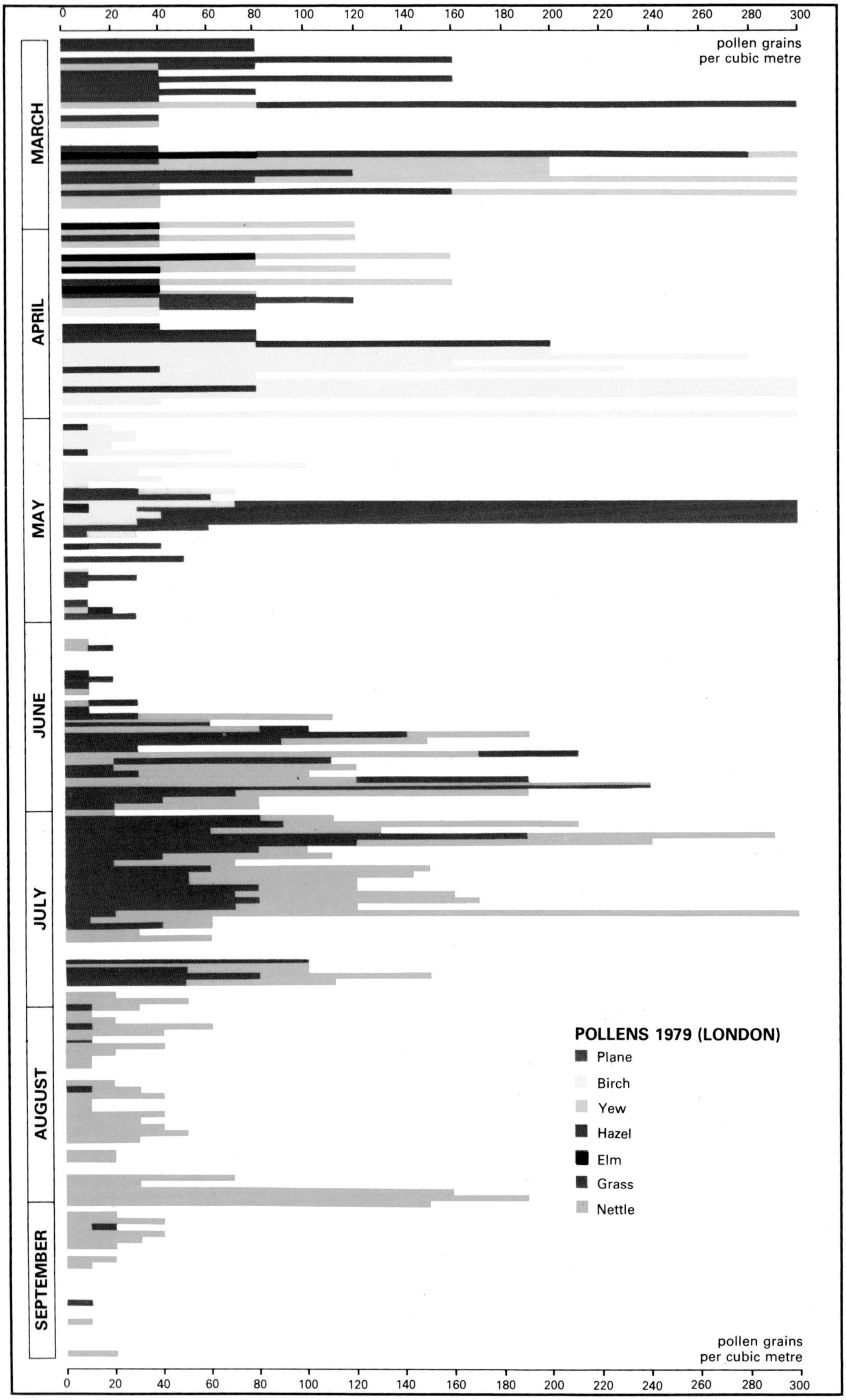

MARCH

APRIL

MAY

JUNE

JULY

AUGUST

SEPTEMBER

POLLENS 1979 (LONDON)
- Plane
- Birch
- Yew
- Hazel
- Elm
- Grass
- Nettle

pollen grains
per cubic metre

22 The pollen count in London in 1979—a typical year. The sticky plate is examined after a collection period of 24 hours and the pollen count expressed as 'grains per cubic metre'. A count of 50 pollen grains per cubic metre may cause discomfort to sensitized individuals, but responses vary; and the grass pollen count does not differentiate between the many different grasses to which an individual may react.

23 The house dust mite—*Dermatophagoides pteronyssinus*. This species and *D. farinae* are most commonly responsible for mite-related symptoms, though other mites have also been implicated, especially in an agricultural setting. They cause symptoms through allergens excreted in their faeces. The faecal particles are about 20 μm in diameter—about the same size as a pollen grain.

Dust mites are commonest in moist, temperate environments. They feed on shed scales of human and animal skin, and thus commonly infest mattresses, pillows, carpets and soft furnishings. They are about 0.5 mm in length and invisible to the naked eye.

In the northern hemisphere mite-induced symptoms are often most severe between November and January, when mite-counts are at their highest; but dust mite allergy is a potent cause of perennial rhinitis and asthma, and possibly also of eczema.

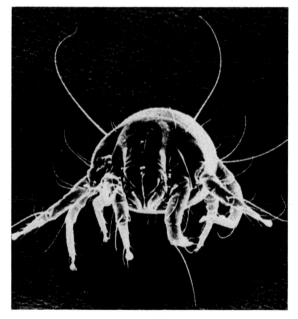

23

DUST PRECAUTIONS

The most important sources of house-dust are soft furnishings and household bedding, particularly mattresses. Your bedroom must be made as dust-free as possible, because you spend more time in this room than any other.

1 All pillows and eiderdowns in the bedroom must be filled with a synthetic material, such as foam rubber or terylene. Feathers, flock or kapok filled pillows and eiderdowns should be removed from the room completely and replaced. This also applies to duvets.

2 On a sunny, warm day when you are out of the house a friend should take your mattress outside into the open air and beat it thoroughly, followed by thorough vacuuming. The mattress should then be covered with a plastic cover, or alternatively vacuum cleaned every week.

3 Change and wash your pillow cases, sheets and underblanket every week and sponge the plastic mattress cover or vacuum clean the mattress at the same time.

4 There is a risk of becoming allergic to animals if you are not already. Animals should not be permitted to sit on sofas, armchairs or other soft furnishings. No animals, birds or other pets should be allowed in the bedroom at any time nor should they be allowed, if possible, in the rooms you spend most of your time in.

These are the most important measures. In addition, we suggest:

● If you have to do your own vacuum cleaning, use disposable paper bags. Never empty one out yourself.

● Do not use dustpan and brushes or brooms. Do not shake carpets and rugs. Never beat any upholstered furniture.

● Dusting must always be done with damp or oiled cloths and mops.

24 Dust precautions. Controlling house dust can sometimes be useful as a diagnostic procedure; and it is certainly worth trying as a preventive tool in those with dust mite allergy. A patient 'handout' of this kind can be very helpful.

Special attention should be paid to the bedroom. A plastic mattress cover is very effective in reducing the mite population, but may prove uncomfortable. Synthetic materials in mattresses, bedding, pillows, carpets, etc. are preferable to mite-supporting materials such as feather, animal hair, flock or kapok.

It is always wise to banish domestic animals from the bedroom. Even where they do not directly cause allergic symptoms, their presence will increase the amount of dust on which the mites can live.

3 ALLERGIC SKIN DISORDERS

A number of skin disorders, some of which have systemic manifestations, can be explained by Gell and Coombs' types I, II, III or IV allergic reactivity (see Table 9), but it is increasingly clear that some dermatological disorders are caused by a complex interplay of more than one mechanism.

'Allergic' skin disorders such as urticaria and eczema can also be related to other endogenous or exogenous factors. They may develop after prolonged exposure of the immune system to the allergen (an induction period). An acquired specific alteration in the capacity to react to antigen is fundamental to the mechanism of allergy, and this tendency towards pathological immune reactions may be inherited. A genetic predisposition exists for atopy and for some of the autoimmune diseases.

Table 9. Gell and Coombs' types of mechanisms of skin injury

Immune type	I	II	III	IV
Alternative name	Immediate	Cytotoxic antibody	Antigen - antibody immune - complex	Delayed-type. Cell-mediated
Cells involved	Mast cell Basophil Eosinophil	B or K Macrophage	B Polymorph Platelets	T Macrophage Giant and epithelioid
Immunoglobulin	IgE	IgE; IgM	IgG	-
Clinical disorder:				
Skin	Urticaria Angioedema Atopic eczema	Pemphigus Pemphigoid Dermatitis herpetiformis	Vasculitis Erythema nodosum	Contact dermatitis Photo-allergic dermatitis
Systemic	Asthma Rhinitis Conjunctivitis		Systemic lupus erythematosus Rheumatoid arthritis Serum sickness Behçêt's syndrome	Graft rejection Sarcoidosis
Appropriate investigations	Skin-prick tests Specific serum IgE (RAST)	Immunofluorescence	Circulating immune complexes Complement conversion High ESR Immunofluorescence	Patch tests Lymphocyte transformation Macrophage migration inhibition Cell-mediated cytotoxity

ECZEMA AND DERMATITIS

The terms eczema and dermatitis are best regarded as synonymous. They both refer to a type of skin inflammation with characteristic clinical and histological features. The skin shows a combination of erythema, vesication, weeping and scaling. Eczema may be acute, subacute or chronic. The most commonly used subdivision is:

● Exogenous (or contact) eczema
● Endogenous (or constitutional) eczema.

These can be further subdivided as shown in Table 10.

Table 10. Classification of eczema

Endogenous
   Atopic*
   Seborrhoeic
   Nummular (Discoid)
   Pompholyx (Dishidrotic)
   Varicose/gravitational/stasis

Exogenous
   Primary irritant
   Contact allergic*

Unclassified
   Neurodermatitis/lichen simplex chronicus
   Nodular prurigo
   Juvenile plantar dermatosis

Metabolic and deficiency conditions
   Phenylketonuria
   Wiskoff-Aldrich syndrome
   Anhidrotic ectodermal dysplasia
   Pellagra
   Malabsorption (essential fatty acids)

*Proven immunological mechanisms

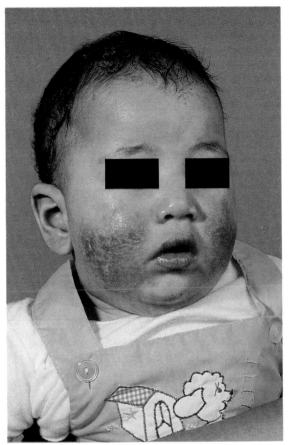

Atopic eczema

Atopy is a genetic predisposition to form excessive IgE antibodies and to develop one or more of a group of disorders which include asthma, hay fever, conjunctivitis and a particular type of eczema. Multiple positive immediate skin-prick tests to commonly tested allergens (see Chapter 2) are commonly present. Defective cell-mediated immunity and fluctuation in the 'in vivo' expression of cell-mediated immunity are also reported.

Atopic eczema affects about 5 per cent of the population, and is a chronic remitting pruritic cutaneous disorder with a strong genetic aetiological component. Seventy per cent of patients have a family history of atopy. Atopic eczema usually begins before the age of six months. The distribution and character of the lesions vary with age, but most patients have generally dry skin throughout life. Fortunately the condition remits spontaneously in 65 per cent of affected children before 10 years of age. Evidence is accumulating that atopic eczema in children may represent a cutaneous manifestation of allergy to a wide variety of environmental allergens including some in food and possibly the house dust mite. A rare complication in a few patients with chronic atopic eczema is the development of cataracts.

25 Infantile atopic eczema. This has a characteristic distribution, affecting the face and neck, as shown in this seven-month-old boy.

26 Atopic eczema. This starts with erythematous and oedematous patches, followed by variable vesiculation and oozing. Scaling erosions and circumscribed lichenification are seen in later stages of the disease. This infant shows how the eczema involves the extensor surfaces.

27 Infantile eczema. This presents in many forms, including seborrhoeic dermatitis and napkin dermatitis. An infant with atopic eczema is often irritable and wakeful, and affected areas may be exacerbated by rubbing.

28 Dennie-Morgan intraorbital folds. These can be seen in this 10-year-old boy with the characteristic facies of atopic eczema. Intense rubbing of the eyes can also produce darkening of the skin around the eyes and even keratoconus.

29 Flexural lichenification and linearity due to excoriation. This develops in both childhood and adult atopic eczema.

26

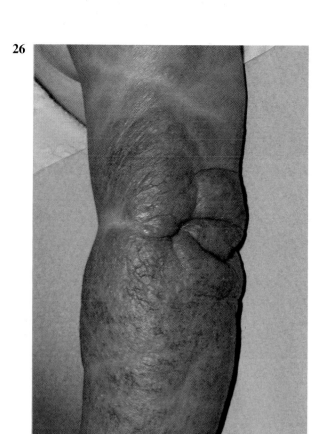

27

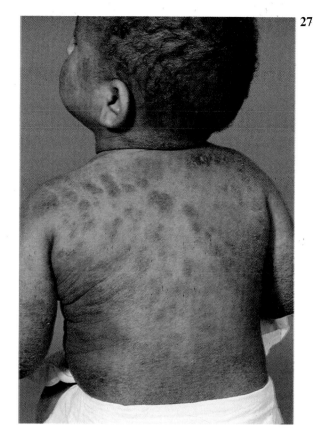

28

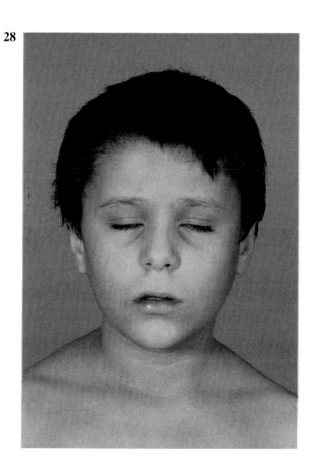

29

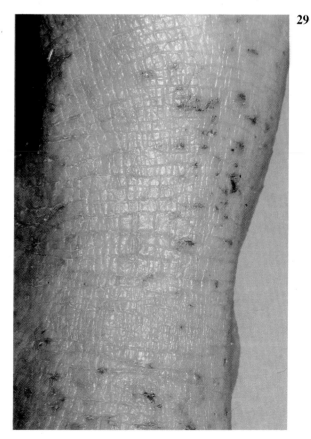

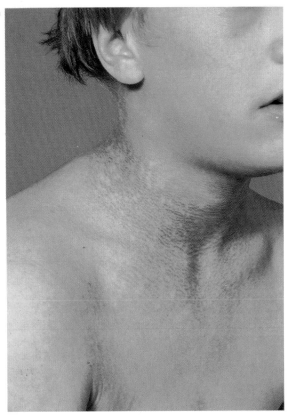

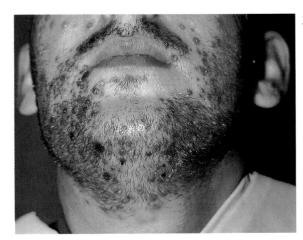

30 Apparent hyperpigmentation. This can occur in atopic eczema, especially over flexures or the neck folds, as a result of severe lichenification.

31 Herpes simplex infection, particularly from cold sores, may severely complicate atopic eczema. This is called Kaposi's varicelliform eruption or eczema herpeticum.

32 Impetiginised eczema. Atopic eczema patients have defective cell-mediated immunity, and are more susceptible not only to viral and fungal infections, but also to bacteria such as *Staphylococcus aureus*.

Seborrhoeic eczema
This type of eczema is usually confined to areas richly populated with sebaceous glands. Perifollicular, erythematous pink or yellow lesions which develop into macular patches appear on the scalp and face, in the retroauricular, pre-sternal, interscapula and intertriginous areas. Typical eczematous changes are seen only occasionally. Increased sebum production and hyperhidrosis provide a base for microbial action and inflammatory changes. In infants, seborrhoeic eczema clears rapidly, but in adults it may be chronic.

32

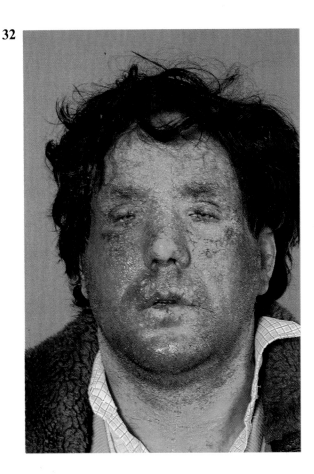

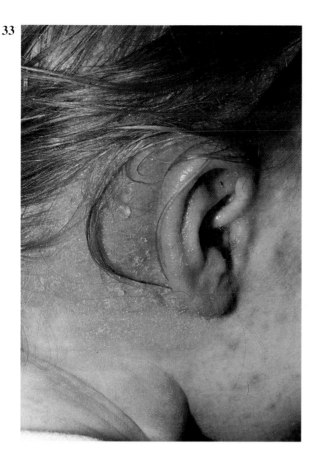

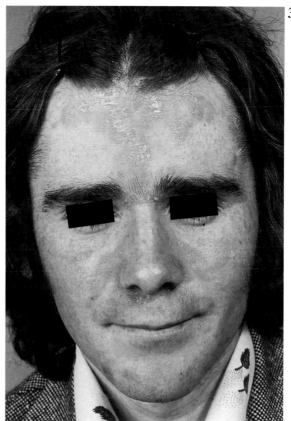

33 Infantile seborrhoeic dermatitis. This often affects the scalp severely, with the presence of erythema and yellow adherent scales. Despite the florid eruption, the infant is well and the condition is self-limiting.

34 Seborrhoeic dermatitis, unrelated to the infantile type, is found chiefly in adult males, as in this 21-year-old. The face is commonly affected.

35 Asymptomatic seborrhoeic dermatitis in a 42-year-old man. Seborrhoeic dermatitis is commonly asymptomatic with red-yellow lesions affecting the pre-sternal area, the nasolabial folds and the external ear. It may be very persistent.

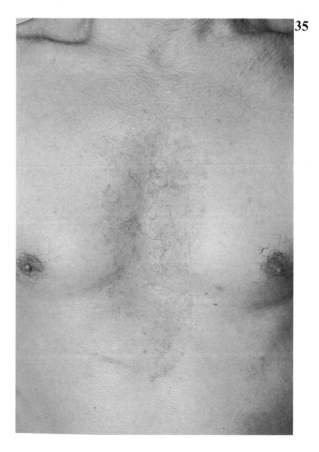

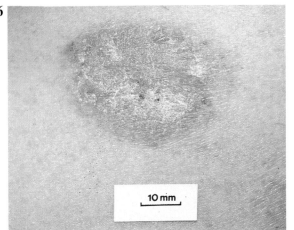

Nummular eczema

This is characterised by pruritic, coin-like, oozing patches, frequently located on the extensor surfaces, and commonest in middle-aged males. In patients with an atopic history, it may be considered as an exudative form of neurodermatitis in contrast to the dry form, which is called lichen simplex.

36 Nummular or discoid eczema in a 39-year-old man. The lesions are subacute, with erythema, mild oedema and some vesiculation. The aetiology is unknown and secondary infection is common.

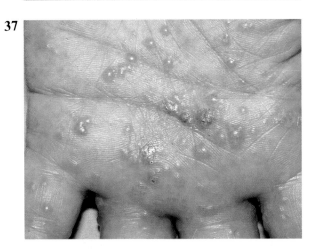

Pompholyx

This variant of eczema can be unpleasant. Recurrent vesicles or bullae affect the palms, fingers and/or soles of adults. It is characterised by remissions and relapses, which are sometimes provoked by heat, emotional stress or an active fungal infection of the feet. There have been reports that ingestion of small amounts of nickel in susceptible patients may trigger an attack.

37 Pompholyx of the hand (cheiropompholyx), showing characteristic vesicles.

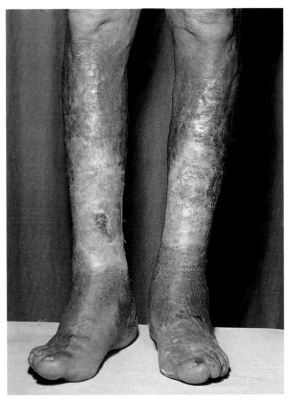

Stasis eczema

Stasis eczema presents as a chronic condition, affecting the lower legs of middle-aged and elderly patients. It is often accompanied by venous insufficiency, with obvious varicose veins, oedema, haemosiderin deposition and lipodermatosclerosis. The venous insufficiency may lead to ulcer formation. Topical medicaments used in venous ulceration can aggravate the condition by causing contact allergic eczema in addition to the underlying stasis eczema.

38 Stasis eczema. This is commonly seen in elderly females, in association with venous insufficiency or frank ulceration. This 68-year-old woman's legs also show marked pigmentation due to haemosiderin deposition.

Neurodermatitis

Neurodermatitis or lichen simplex chronicus usually presents with a single, fixed, lichenified plaque, which is perpetuated by repeated rubbing or scratching as a habit or as a response to stress. Favourite sites are the nape of neck in women, the legs in men, and the anogenital area in both sexes. Lesions tend to be chronic.

Irritant eczema

Irritants account for the majority of industrial eczema cases and the resulting work loss. Strong irritants are usually easy to identify, but prolonged exposure, sometimes over a period of years, is needed for weak irritants to cause eczema. The commonest site of irritant eczema is the hands, and culprit substances include detergents, alkalis, solvents, cutting oils and abrasive dusts.

Napkin dermatitis is due to irritant ammonical urine and faeces, which tend to spare the skin folds. Psoralens in plants or perfumes can cause photodermatitis. This reaction is not an allergic one, though some light-induced eczemas are due to type IV hypersensitivity.

Allergic contact eczema

Allergic contact eczema is caused by delayed cutaneous hypersensitivity to environmental allergens (type IV) which persists indefinitely once established. It is diagnosed from the history of onset following exposure to a sensitising agent and an appropriate distribution of lesions. Secondary spread of lesions may, however, occur and it is not always easy to track down the responsible allergen. Questioning should cover both occupational and domestic exposure.

Diagnosis is confirmed by patch testing with appropriate allergens (see Chapter 2). Some common sensitising agents and their sources are shown in Table 11.

Table 11. Common allergens in contact eczema

Allergen	Source
Nickel	Jewellery, jean studs, bra clips
Balsam of Peru	Perfumes, citrus fruits
Dichromate	Cement, leather, matches
Paraphenylene-diamine	Hair dyes, clothing
Rubber chemicals	Shoes, clothing, gloves
Colophony	Sticking plaster, collodium
Neomycin	Topical medicaments
Benzocaine	
Parabens	Preservatives in cosmetics and creams
Wood alcohols	Lanolin, cosmetics, creams

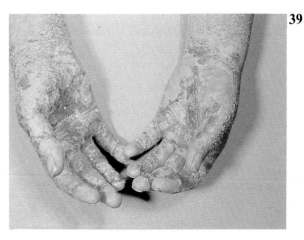

39

39 Irritant eczema, presenting as hand dermatitis in a 39-year-old man. It resulted from exposure to irritant chemicals at work.

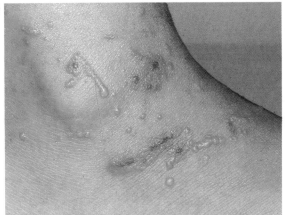

40 Poison ivy dermatitis is a common contact dermatitis in North America. This 15-year-old boy presented with linear eczematous lesions on his ankle.

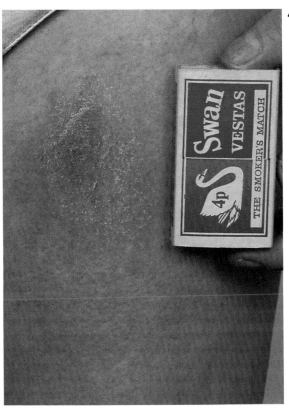

41 Phosphorus sequisulphide sensitivity and its source. This 53-year-old man had eczema of the face, hands and thigh, which resulted from his sensitivity to the chemical in red-tipped matches. Note the relationship of the high dermatitis to the area of the trouser pocket in which he carried the matches.

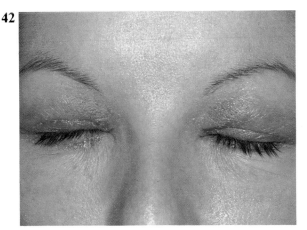

42 Blepharitis. Characterised by redness and swelling of the eye lid margins, this can be due to contact allergic dermatitis to eye make-up, as in this 22-year-old-woman.

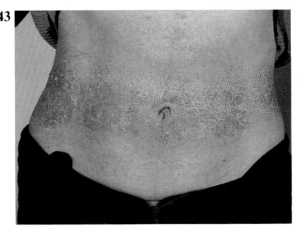

43 Rubber contact allergy. This can sometimes be diagnosed on distribution, as shown in this 30-year-old woman who became sensitive to the rubber in her girdle.

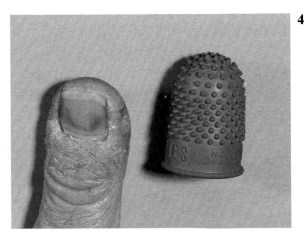

44 Finger stall dermatitis. Another example of contact allergy to rubber.

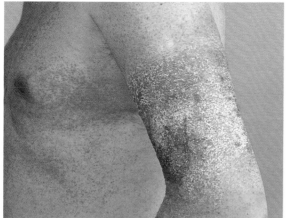

45 Rubber contact allergy in a 51-year-old man. This followed repeated use of a sphygmomanometer cuff for blood pressure measurement.

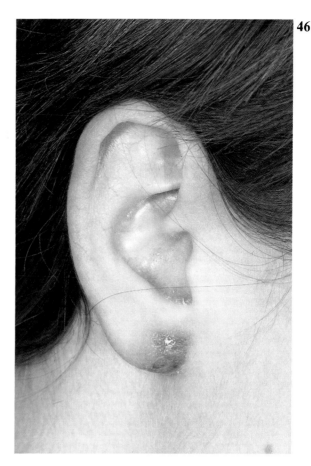

46 Contact allergic dermatitis to nickel. This affects 10 per cent of European women. Nickel is a commonly used metal, found in jewellery such as rings, necklaces and ear-rings. Nickel in ear-rings gave rise to ear lobe eczema in this young woman.

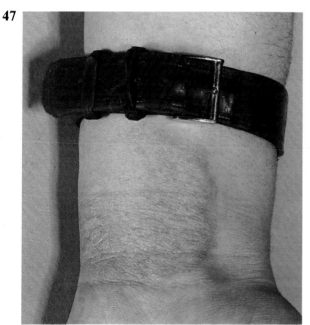

47 Nickel contact allergy. Another example, showing a reaction to nickel in the buckle of a wrist watch strap.

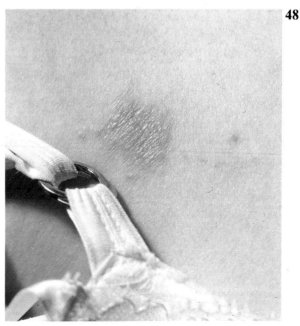

48 Nickel contact allergy. This is commonly due to nickel in the metal parts of clothes.

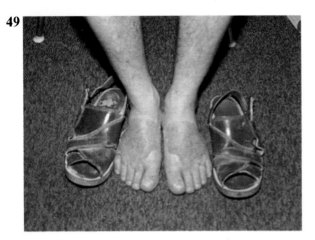

49 **Chromium contact allergy presented as dermatitis of the foot in this 50-year-old man.** Note the relationship of the dermatitis to his sandals. Chromium is used as a tanning agent in curing leather.

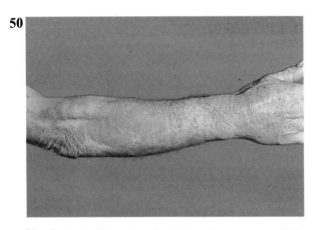

50 **Contact allergy to plants is quite common.** This 73-year-old gardener became sensitised to chrysanthemums. The eczema affects his hands and forearms.

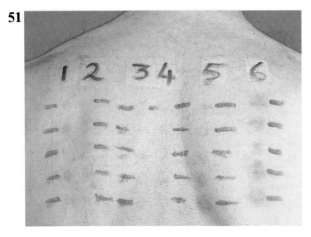

51 **Patch test of the gardener in 50.** This confirmed that he was sensitive to all the types of chrysanthemums which he grew.

Management of eczema

Individual types of eczema need investigation and treatment which differ in detail, but which are based upon similar general principles. Differential diagnoses in chronic cases should include fungal infection, psoriasis and Bowen's disease.

Acute weeping eczema is treated by soaking in a 1:10,000 solution of potassium permanganate. Patients should avoid soap and use lubricants liberally. Emollients in the form of emulsifying ointment baths and aqueous cream are essential. Stabilised urea preparations may be helpful. In severe cases of widespread bacterial infection, systemic antibiotics may be required. In more chronic cases, particularly of atopic eczema, oral antihistamines or occlusive bandages may relieve pruritis. Aggravating factors such as woollen clothes or heat should be avoided. Any specific food allergens in atopics, particularly in children, should be excluded from the diet (see Chapter 8).

Contact allergens should be suspected when there is a poor response to treatment and identified by patch testing. Other treatment for contact eczema is similar to that for atopic eczema. In seborrhoeic eczema, 2 per cent sulphur and 2 per cent salicylic acid in aqueous cream is useful and often avoids the need for topical steroids.

URTICARIA

Urticaria is common, and usually presents as acute, transient but recurrent, pruritic, erythematous cutaneous swellings due to fluid transfer from the vasculature to the dermis. It is often minor (weals) but rarely severe and life threatening, affecting the laryngeal area (as in severe angioedema). Similar reactions can occur in other organs, e.g. gastrointestinal tract, joints and bronchi. In many cases, the lesions are self-limiting.

In 75 per cent of all chronic urticaria the aetiology is unknown, though there are several recognised causes for acute cases. Both immunological and non-immunological factors may precipitate urticaria (see Table 12).

Diagnosis is often self evident, and a careful history often reveals an obvious cause. Painful persistent lesions should raise the possibility of urticarial vasculitis. The majority of chronic cases of urticaria yield negative results on investigation and must be treated on a symptomatic basis with antihistamines. In some cases an elemination diet may prove useful (see Chapter 8). Anaphylactic reactions may require treatment with subcutaneous adrenalin and even immediate cardiopulmonary resuscitation in severe cases.

Table 12. Classification of urticaria

Immunologic	Aetiology
IgE dependent	Atopic Specific antigen sensitivity, e.g. food, worms Physical, e.g. dermographism, pressure, heat, water, cold, sunlight, cholinergic*
Complement-mediated	Hereditary angiodema, e.g. C_1 esterase inhibitor deficiency Acquired, e.g. lymphoma Autoimmune

Non-immunologic	Aetiology
Substances which directly stimulate mast cell degranulation	Drugs, e.g. opiates, quinine, chlortetracycline, aspirin Chemicals, e.g. dextran, azo-dyes, benzoates Foods, e.g. egg white, strawberries and shell fish
Histamine-containing foods	e.g. some cheeses, mackerel and tuna fish
Physical agents and cholinergic effects*	

*Most, but not all, physical and cholingeric effects are probably non-immunologic in mechanism.

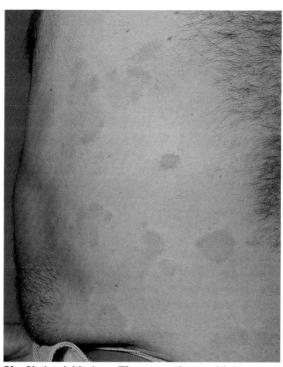

52 Urticarial lesions. These are often multiple, transient, erythematous weals or plaques, which itch but disappear within 24 hours, as happened in this 41-year-old man. Failure to remit within 24 hours should alert the clinician to the possibility of vasculitis.

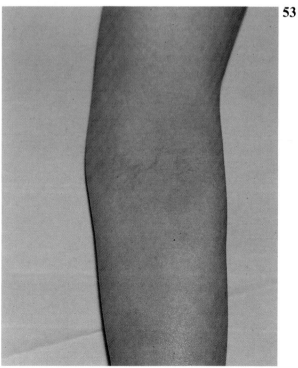

53 Cholinergic urticaria. This occurred in this susceptible individual following an increase in core body temperature resulting from a hot bath or exercise.

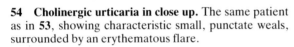

54 **Cholinergic urticaria in close up.** The same patient as in **53**, showing characteristic small, punctate weals, surrounded by an erythematous flare.

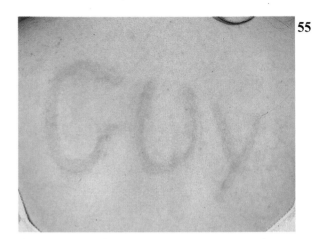

55 **Dermographism is a form of urticaria in which the patient responds to anything more than a very light touch with a weal and flare reaction.** This can be simply tested with firm finger pressure as shown in this patient from a well-known London teaching hospital.

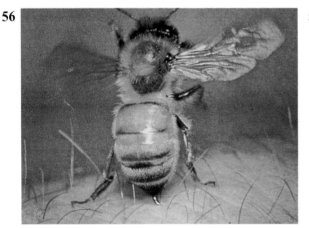

56 **Bee sting allergy is an important cause of urticaria and of life-threatening angioedema and anaphylaxis.** Other stinging insects such as wasps may cause similar problems in sensitised patients.

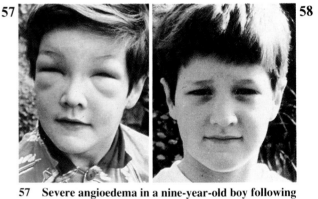

57 **Severe angioedema in a nine-year-old boy following a bee sting.** The patient required immediate treatment with adrenalin to overcome his anaphylactic response.
58 **Bee sting allergy.** The same patient as in **57** without angioedema. Encouraging developments in desensitisation therapy may prevent further severe reactions in patients with insect venom.

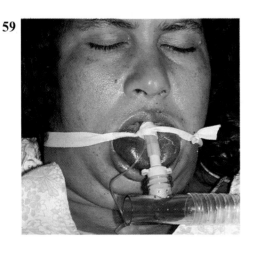

59 **Severe angioedema in a 43-year-old woman.** She required endotracheal intubation to overcome laryngeal obstruction. Note the oedema of her mouth and face. This patient had a family history of similar problems, and she was subsequently found to have a rare C_1 esterase inhibitor deficiency. This form of urticaria is thus complement mediated.

60

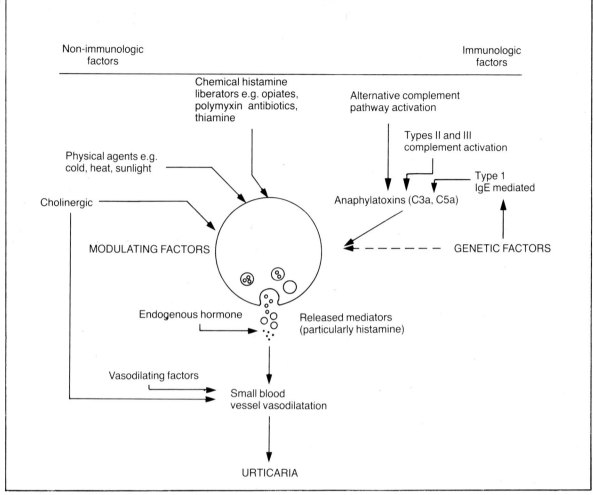

Non-immunologic factors

Immunologic factors

Chemical histamine liberators e.g. opiates, polymyxin antibiotics, thiamine

Alternative complement pathway activation

Types II and III complement activation

Physical agents e.g. cold, heat, sunlight

Type 1 IgE mediated

Cholinergic

Anaphylatoxins (C3a, C5a)

MODULATING FACTORS

GENETIC FACTORS

Endogenous hormone

Released mediators (particularly histamine)

Vasodilating factors

Small blood vessel vasodilatation

URTICARIA

60 The pathophysiology of urticaria. Mast cells can be stimulated to release mediators by various immunological and nonimmunologic factors. Histamine is often the mediator responsible for the cutaneous vascular changes seen in urticaria, but many other naturally occurring substances may be involved. IgE antibodies are often, but not always, involved in mast cell degranulation.

Table 13. Investigations in chronic persistent urticaria

Full blood count and blood film
Erythrocyte sedimentation rate
Liver function tests
Chest xray, Sinus xrays
Examination of fresh stools for parasites
Examination of urine for bacteria
Complement screen, including C_1 esterase inhibitor
Autoantibodies
Hepatitis B surface antigen

IMMUNO-BULLOUS DISORDERS

Pemphigus

Pemphigus vulgaris is one of four varieties of pemphigus, the others being pemphigus vegetans, pemphigus folliaceus and pemphigus erythematosus. Immunological studies show that it is an autoimmune disorder. It is commoner in Jews, and affects both sexes equally. Cutaneous and circulating antibody is directed to intercellular substance of the epidermis. The titre of this antibody correlates with disease activity. Blisters may develop on both mucous membranes and skin. Skin biopsy shows an intraepidermal blister and direct immunofluorescence confirms tissue-fixed intercellular IgG antibody in the epidermis. The indirect test for circulating antibody gives a similar result, but requires substrate tissue, e.g. primate oesophagus or human vaginal mucosa. Following incubation with the patient's serum, fluorescein-labelled antibody to IgG and complement is applied. The serum can be diluted and quantified.

Pemphigus should be treated with high-dose systemic steroids and antibiotics. In untreated pemphigus, secondary infection and fluid and electrolyte imbalance can be fatal. Long-term treatment with steroids or immunosuppressive drugs is often necessary.

61
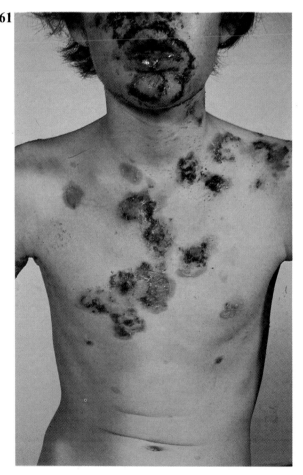

62
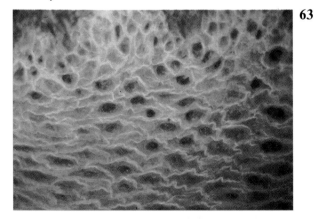

62 Pemphigus vulgaris blisters are thin and painful with an intraepidermal split. They often become secondarily infected.

63
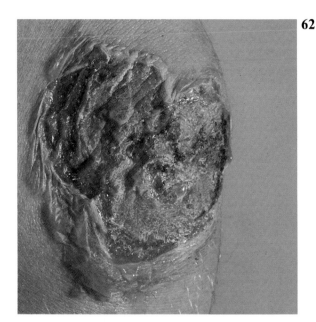

61 Pemphigus vulgaris. This often begins insidiously, as happened in this 13-year-old boy. In addition to the skin lesions, raw areas and shallow erosions often occur on mucous membranes, especially in the mouth.

63 Direct immunofluorescence in pemphigus vulgaris, showing intercellular epidermal deposition of IgG. C_3 and occasionally IgM may also be deposited.

Pemphigoid

Pemphigoid, sometimes termed 'bullous pemphigoid' to distinguish it from cicatricial pemphigoid, usually affects patients over 60 years of age. The blister is sub-epidermal (between dermis and epidermis). As with pemphigus, tissue-fixed and circulating autoantibodies have been demonstrated, suggesting that the disease may have an auto-immune pathogenesis. Immunoglobulin and complement are found in a linear band at the dermoepidermal junction. Blisters occur on proximal parts of the limbs on an eczematous base. These can bleed spontaneously and may become infected, requiring systemic antibiotic therapy. Oral lesions are rarer than in pemphigus. Immunosuppressives including large doses of systemic steroids are necessary, but they may usually be reduced after two or three years.

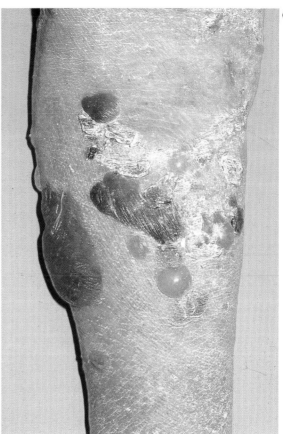

65   Pemphigoid. This 89-year-old patient's blisters became haemorrhagic, as often occurs.

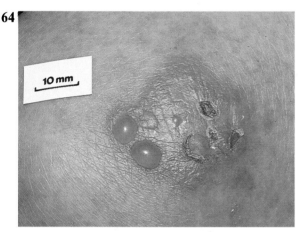

64   Pemphigoid blisters in an 88-year-old woman. There is debate about a possible association between this condition and internal malignancy, and this patient was found subsequently to have carcinoma of the colon.

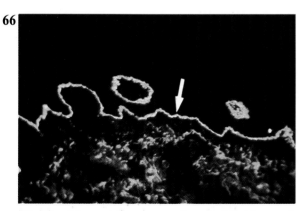

66   Direct immunofluorescence in pemphigoid reveals IgG deposition in the basement membrane (arrow) in perilesional skin biopsies. Granular deposition of C_3 is often observed.

Herpes gestationis

Herpes gestationis is a rare disease of pregnancy, which tends to recur in successive pregnancies. Classically, it resembles bullous pemphigoid in its appearance, but at the other end of the clinical spectrum it merges into other eruptions of pregnancy, especially toxic urticated erythemas. The most common finding on direct immunofluorescence of perilesional skin is linear deposition of C_3 along the basement membrane zone. In 40 per cent of patients, IgG is also found at the dermo-epidermal junction. In fewer patients than in bullous pemphigoid, complement fixing IgG autoantibodies, the 'HG factor' can be isolated. There are several reports of increased fetal death rate and transient rashes and antibodies in the baby. In severe cases this condition should be treated with systemic corticosteroids.

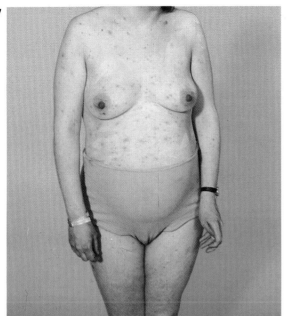

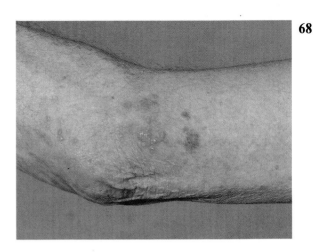

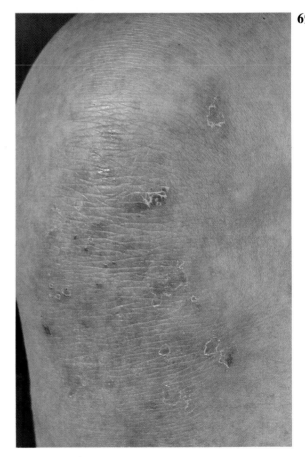

67   Herpes gestationis. This is a rare pruritic eruption occurring during pregnancy and the puerperium. Vesicles and bullae associated with patchy erythema occur as in this 33-year-old woman.

Dermatitis herpetiformis

Dermatitis herpetiformis is an intensely pruritic skin condition, associated with deposition of IgA in dermal papillae, and with gluten-sensitive enteropathy. Patients usually present in the third and fourth decade, and males are more commonly affected than females. The blisters are sub-epidermal and small compared with the larger lesions of bullous pemphigoid. No circulating antibody has yet been consistently found in dermatitis herpetiformis patients, but direct im-munofluorescence of the skin is diagnostic.

Most patients will not have overt symptoms or signs of malabsorption, but even so a jejunal biopsy should be performed to identify sub-total villous atrophy. If this is present, it should be treated with a gluten-free diet. These lesions respond within 24-48 hours to dapsone and to a gluten-free diet over two or three years.

Linear IgA dermatosis

This affects a small sub-group of patients clinically diagnosed as having dermatitis herpetiformis, but found to have a linear rather than a granular pattern of IgA on immunofluoresc-ence. The condition seems to differ in some respects from dermatitis herpetiformis. Gluten enteropathy seems to be less common, and the increased incidence of HLA B8 and DW3 does not occur.

68, 69 and 70   Dermatitis herpetiformis is an intensely pruritic, subepidermal blistering condition, which commonly affects the elbows, scapula areas, buttocks and scalp. The vesicles are much smaller than those in bullous pemphigoid.

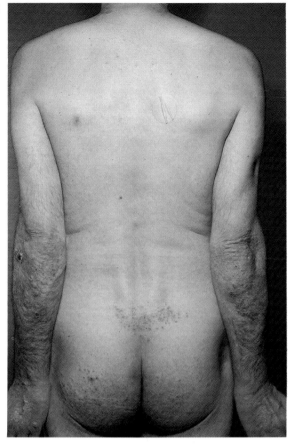

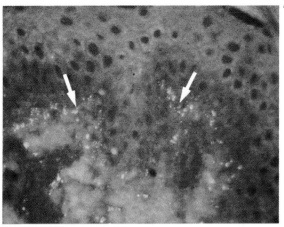

71 Immunofluorescence in dermatitis herpetiformis. This reveals IgA deposition in the papillary dermis (arrows) in perilesional skin.

Table 14. The differential diagnosis of immuno-bullous disorders

	Site	History	Histology	Immunology	Other tests
Pemphigus	Mucous membranes and trunk	Insidious onset	Intraepidermal blister	Direct IgG, C_3 Circulating IgG	
Pemphigoid	Upper arms and thighs	Blisters on eczematous base	Subepidermal blister	Fixed IgG and C_3 at dermoepidermal junction Circulating IgG	
Dermatitis herpetiformis	Scalp, scapula area, elbows, buttocks	Pruritus	Subepidermal blister	IgA in papillary dermis	Sub-total villous atrophy on jejunal biopsy

4 ALLERGY TO DRUGS

Adverse effects resulting from drug administration are an increasingly well-recognised problem. Many adverse reactions can be prevented by adhering rigidly to the recommended dose of drug, by considering and avoiding drug interactions with other drugs or diseases and by careful clinical monitoring. Idiosyncratic reactions may still occur, however, as these are by their nature unpredictable.

Idiosyncratic reactions to drugs are not necessarily 'allergic' as the drug often does not act as an antigen, and, though the end result may resemble an allergic reaction, the mechanisms involved in the host are 'chemical' rather than truly allergic in nature.

The term 'allergic drug reaction' should be reserved for those responses in which the drug is acting as an allergen and inducing a hypersensitivity state. This may produce a wide spectrum of hypersensitivity reactions. Skin rashes are the commonest manifestation of allergy to drugs, but other organ systems may be affected, and the most serious immediate consequence of a true allergic drug reaction is gross angioedema and anaphylaxis. Other drugs may lead to the development of a more chronic immune disorder such as systemic lupus erythematosus (see page 97).

The diagnosis of allergy to a drug is usually based on clinical observations and appropriate detective work (see Tables 15 and 16).

Table 15.   Clinical criteria for drug allergy

- The observed manifestations do not resemble the pharmacological action of the drug.

- The reactions are generally similar to those which may occur with other allergens.

- An induction period, commonly 7-10 days, is required upon initial exposure to the drug.

- The reaction may be reproduced by cross-reacting chemical structures

- The reaction may be reproduced by minute doses of the drug.

- Blood and/or tissue eosinophilia may be present.

- Discontinuation of the drug results in resolution of the reaction.

- The allergic reaction occurs in a minority of patients receiving the drug.

Table 16.   Factors influencing the development of drug allergy

Drug factors	Nature of drug Cross-sensitization Route of administration Degree of exposure
Host factors	Age and sex Genetic factors Previous drug reactions Underlying diseases

---

Table 17.   Drugs frequently implicated in allergic drug reactions

- Aspirin
- NSAIDs
- Penicillins
- Sulphonamides
- Antituberculous drugs
- Nitrofurans
- Antimalarials
- Griseofulvin
- Hypnotics
- Anticonvulsants
- Anaesthetic agents
- Muscle relaxants
- Tranquillizers
- Antihypertensives
- Antiarrhythmics
- Iodinated contrast media
- Antisera and vaccines
- Organ extracts, e.g. insulin, ACTH
- Heavy metals
- Allopurinol
- Penicillamine
- Antithyroid drugs

Table 18. Differences between non-allergic and allergic drug reactions

Difference	Non-allergic	Allergic
Quantities required to provoke reaction	Large	Minute
Cumulative effect	Often necessary	Usually none
Relationship between allergic effect and pharmacological action	Often present	No connection
Same effect reproduced by pharmacologically different chemicals	Rare	Common
Clinical picture	Uniform	Varied

Table 19. Clinical manifestations of drug allergy

Generalised or multisystem involvement
  Anaphylaxis
  Serum-sickness-like reactions
  Drug fever
  Systemic lupus erythematosus-like reactions
  Vasculitis, e.g. Henoch-Schönlein purpura

Reactions predominantly involving one organ system
  Dermatological
    exanthematous (50 per cent)
    urticaria/angioedema (25 per cent)
    contact dermatitis
    fixed drug eruption
    erythema multiforme-like, including
      Stevens-Johnson syndrome
    exfoliative dermatitis
    photosensitivity
    vasculitis
    erythema nodosum
    toxic epidermal necrolysis
    erythematosquamous eruption

Respiratory
  asthma
  hypersensitivity pneumonia
  pulmonary infiltrate with eosinophilia
  vasculitis

Haematological
  cytopenias
  eosinophilia

Hepatic cholestasis
  hepatocellular damage

Renal
  glomerulitis
  interstitial nephritis
  nephrotic syndrome

RE system
  lymphadenopathy

Neurological
  convulsions
  encephalopathy

Table 20. Features of phototoxic and photoallergic reactions

	Phototoxic	Photoallergic
Incidence	Common	Uncommon
Clinical features	Erythematous	Eczematous
Onset after exposure	4-8 hours	12-24 hours
Rash occurs away from exposure site	No	Yes
Following first exposure	Can produce reaction	No reaction unless previous sensitization period of days to months
Drug dosage	Dose related	Dose independent
Immunological mechanism	None	T cell-mediated

Table 21.   Drugs commonly implicated in photosensitivity reactions

	Phototoxic	**Photoallergic**
Topical	Coal tar derivatives e.g. dithranol Psoralens Furocoumarins	Halogenated salicylamides
Systemic	Demeclocycline Doxycycline Chlorpromazine (occasionally)	Phenothiazines Sulphonamides Griseofulvin

Table 22.   Medication often overlooked[*]

- Aspirin and other analgesics
- Nose drops
- Cold 'cures'
- Sedatives
- Laxatives
- Antibiotics
- Tonics
- Contraceptives
- Ointments
- Douches
- Suppositories
- Lozenges
- Dysmenorrhoea treatment

[*]i.e. Considered unimportant by the patient. The doctor should specifically ask about each medication.

Management of allergy to drugs

Once a probable allergic reaction to a drug has been identified, the suspected drug should be withdrawn from the patient. It may often be necessary to withdraw more than one drug as part of the diagnostic process.

The manifestations of the allergic reaction may require treatment in their own right, and anaphylactic reactions will need immediate treatment with subcutaneous or intramuscular adrenaline. Antihistamines may be helpful in pruritic eruptions, and systemic steroids may be needed for generalised reactions such as exfoliative dermatitis or the Stevens-Johnson syndrome. Skin involvement often responds to soothing topical therapy such as a simple calamine lotion or 2 per cent menthol in calamine cream.

Skin-prick tests for drug allergy are hazardous and neither they nor *in vitro* tests can be interpreted clearly in every case. Patch tests have a limited value in eczematous eruptions where tropical therapy is a possible cause, but no other uses in drug allergy.

Once true allergy to a drug has been established, further administration of that drug or other cross-reacting drugs should be avoided unless no other alternatives are available. It is sometimes possible to desensitize a patient to a drug by giving repeated doses under close supervision in hospital, but the effect of this manoeuvre is short-lived unless drug administration is subsequently continuous, so this manoeuvre is only applicable where long-term treatment with the culprit drug is required.

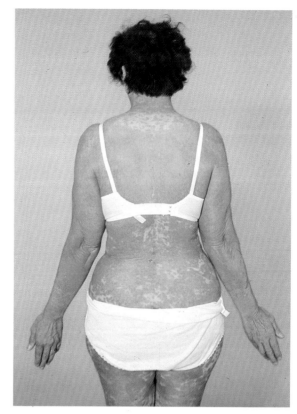

72

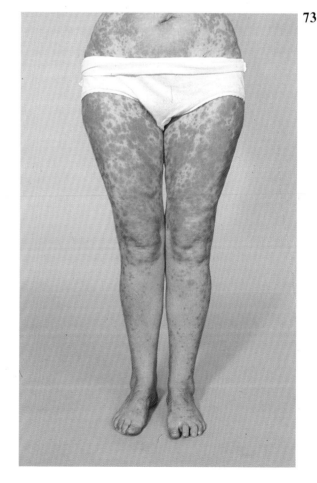

73

72 and 73 Ampicillin rash often presents as a symmetrical erythematous maculopapular eruption, as seen in this 65-year-old woman. This patient seems to have a true allergy to penicillins, but ampicillin drug eruptions are frequently seen in patients with infectious mononucleosis due to the EB virus. In that setting, the rash seems to result from a non-allergic interaction between the drug and the disease.

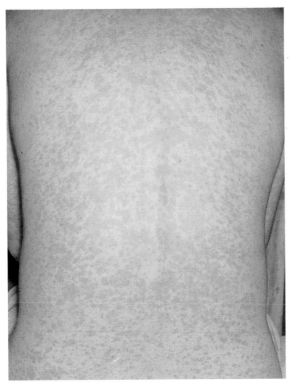

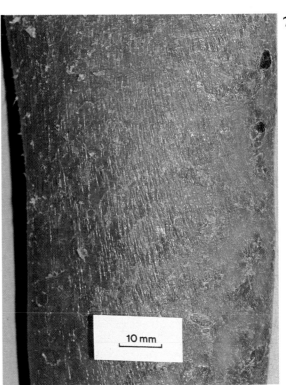

74 A morbilliform eruption in a patient treated with cotrimoxazole. The offending agent here is usually the sulphonamide component, and rashes are much less frequent when trimethoprim is used without sulphonamide. Similar rashes may occur when other sulphonamides are administered.

75 Exfoliative dermatitis is a severe complication of drug sensitivity. This 25-year-old African man developed generalised exfoliative dermatitis following cotrimoxazole therapy.

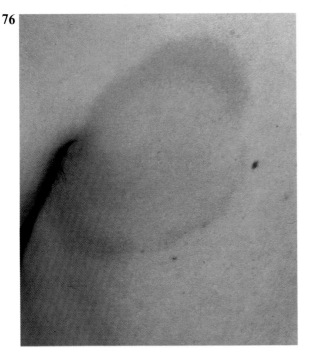

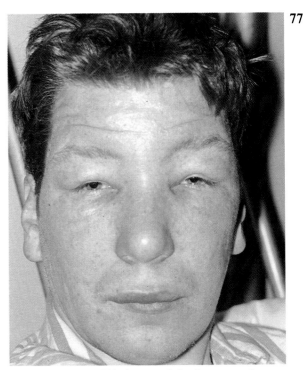

76 Urticaria. This is a common presentation of sensitivity to penicillins—in this case amoxycillin in a 24-year-old man (see also page 38)

77 Angioedema. This is potentially dangerous, but not uncommon following penicillin ingestion—as in this 26-year-old man.

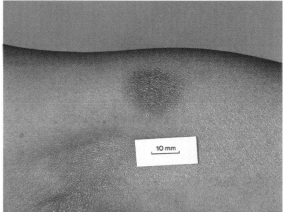

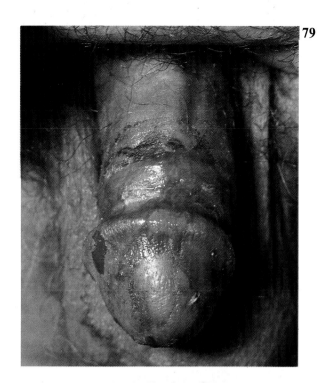

78 A fixed drug eruption, so called because the lesion recurs at the same site after each administration of the causative drug. A common cause is phenolphthalein, found in various proprietary laxative preparations—as here in a 44-year-old Chinese woman. Fixed drug reactions are often misdiagnosed as they are so localised and may present as bullae.

79 Another fixed drug eruption, again due to phenolphthalein. Here it has caused lesions on the genitalia of a 30-year-old man.

80

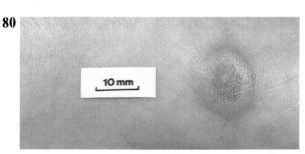

80 Erythema multiforme has a characteristic appearance. This 33-year-old woman was allergic to sulphonamides.

81

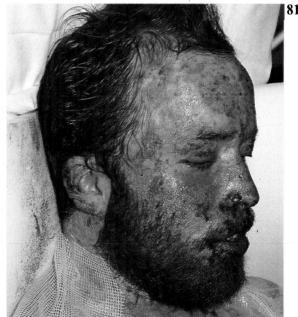

81 Stevens-Johnson syndrome is widespread, severe erythema multiforme with oral, genital and conjunctival involvement.

82

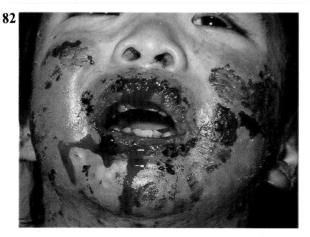

82 Stevens-Johnson syndrome is potentially fatal. In this two-year-old Chinese boy it developed following cotrimoxazole administration.

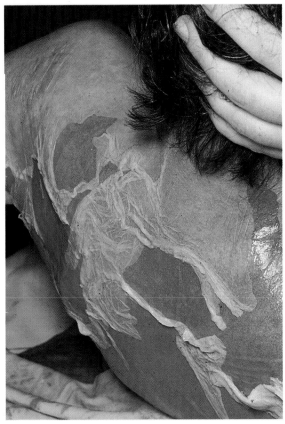

83 Toxic epidermal necrolysis, the 'scalded skin syndrome' in an adult. The commonest cause is drug allergy.

84

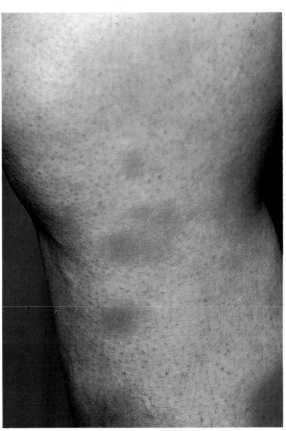

84 Erythema nodosum. This developed on a 45-year-old woman's legs following sulphonamide administration. The lesions are tender and after several weeks they develop a bruised appearance as shown toward the bottom of the picture.

85

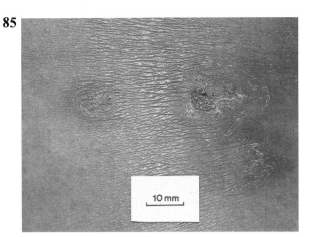

10 mm

85 Gold rashes are not uncommon in rheumatoid patients, and they may persist despite withdrawal of gold therapy.

86

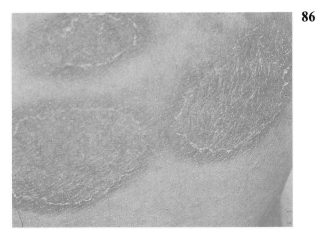

86 Gold sensitivity is more commonly manifest as a psoriasiform eruption.

87

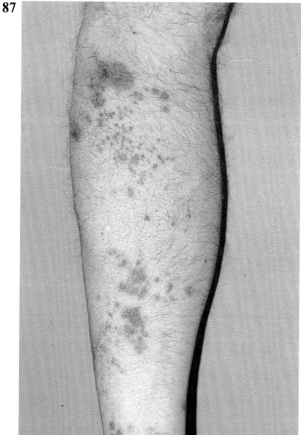

87 **Vasculitis** developed in this 51-year-old man as a result of sensitivity to benzylpenicillin.

88

88 **Vasculitis** must be considered if an eruption is purpuric and palpable. Investigations should include skin biopsy for immunofluorescent studies. This 60-year-old woman developed vasculitis following treatment with a non-steroidal anti-inflammatory drug.

89

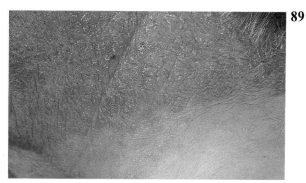

89 **A photoallergic drug reaction** in a 64-year-old man who was taking chlorpromazine. Note how the reaction ceases at the line of his collar. The relationship to light exposure is clear here, but may not always be so obvious.

90

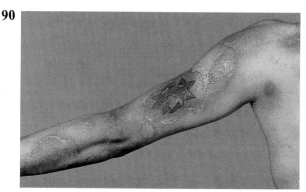

90 **A phototoxic drug eruption,** which developed in this 17-year-old following treatment of his psoriasis with topical coal tar or dithranol, followed by ultraviolet light.

91

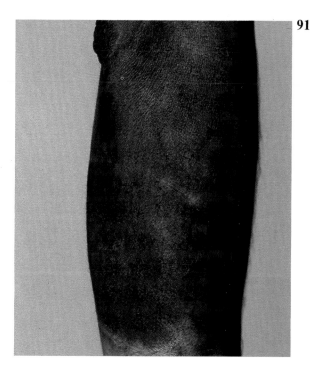

91 **Dithranol staining.** This often develops in treated psoriatic plaques, as on the forearm of this 29-year-old man.

5 ALLERGIC DISORDERS OF THE EYE

The eye presents unique immunological features in that it is relatively isolated from the systemic immune system, and has an efficient local protective system in the structures of the external eye, the tarsal plates and the conjunctiva. The avascularity of the cornea together with the perfect lattice arrangement of the collagen fibrils, surfaced by a five-layer epithelium and lined by a single layer of endothelium, is responsible for its transparency. The lining layers of the eye and its contents, the aqueous humour, vitreous and lens, are kept separate from the immune system by the blood-vitreous and the blood-aqueous barriers. The blood vessels of the retina, ciliary body and iris are characterised by tight junctions between the endothelial cells.

When microbial agents enter the eye, they undergo uninhibited proliferation until a somewhat delayed inflammatory response occurs which itself causes serious visual loss. Special care is taken during ophthalmic surgery to prevent microbial contamination because of the cataclysmic effects that intraocular infections have on vision.

Ocular protection is dependent on the integrity of the structures of the external eye and on first and second lines of defence which are dependent on universal immunological mechanisms (see Table 23).

Although the inflammatory responses of the eye may be comparitively minor when matched against those occurring in other systems, they can have serious consequences. Inflammatory responses of the eye may be provoked by infection or immunological disease.

Table 23. Defence mechanisms in the normal eye

Physical factors
Normal lids, lashes and Meibomian secretions
Normal tarsal and bulbar conjunctiva, and
   corneal epithelial barrier
Normal lid closure (intact VIIth nerve)
Normal sensation (intact Vth nerve)
Normal tear film with intact lipid, aqueous and
   mucus layers

Non-specific immunological mechanisms
Normal content lysozyme, lactoferrin and
   caeruloplasmin in tears
Langerhans' cells in bulbar conjunctiva
Intact complement cascade
Intact polymorphonuclear and macrophage
   migration mechansims

Specific responses
IgA in tears
Specific IgG in corneal stroma
Systemic humoral responses
Systemic cell-mediated responses

Table 24. The manifestations of inflammatory disease in the eye

Inflammatory disease	Clinical manifestation
Conjunctivitis	Inflammatory hyperaemia of tarsal plates Follicular conjunctivitis *(Adenovirus, Chlamydia, trachomatis)* Papillae (hay fever conjunctivitis, vernal catarrh) Chronic scarring (Trachoma) Cicatricial mucous membrane pemphigoid Stevens-Johnson syndrome
Keratitis	Cellular infiltration in corneal stroma Oedema Vascularisation
Scleritis	Nodular or diffuse hyperaemia of deep vessels Necrosis Scleral thinning
Uveitis	Iritis Proteinaceous exudates in anterior chamber (flare) Keratitic precipitates (collections of lymphocytes and plasma cells on corneal endothelium) Cyclitis (inflammation of ciliary body) Inflammatory cells in vitreous Choroiditis (focal inflammation in choroid)
Retinal vasculitis	Haemorrhages, exudates and retinal oedema

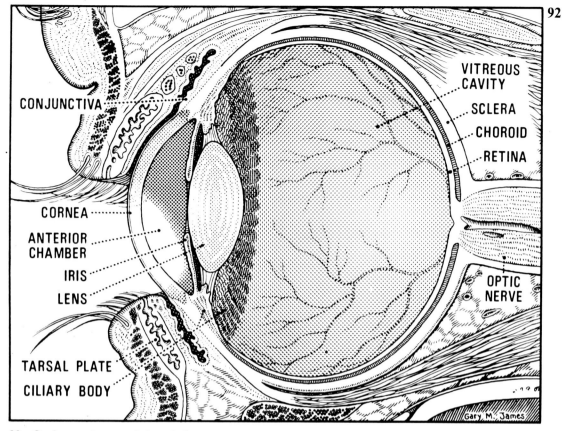

92 Ocular anatomy and targets in immunologically induced disease.

Table 25. Examples of hypersensitivity reactions in the eye

Type I (immediate-type)
Acute allergic conjunctivitis with conjunctival oedema in children
Hay fever conjunctivitis
Vernal keratoconjunctivitis
Atopic conjunctivitis in adults

Type II (cytotoxic-type)
Pemphigus vulgaris
Cicatricial pemphigoid

Type III (complex-mediated)
Scleritis (PAN, RA, SLE, etc)
Erythema multiforme (Major form)

Type IV (cell-mediated, delayed-type)
Contact conjunctivitis
Phlyctenular keratoconjunctivitis
Corneal graft rejection

Mechanism uncertain
Contact lens-associated giant papillary conjunctivitis (GPC)
Peripheral corneal melting syndrome

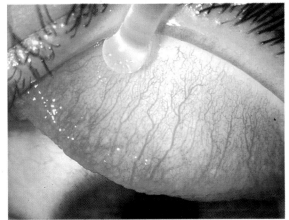

93 **Hay fever conjunctivitis**. The everted upper tarsal plate shows hyperaemia and oedema, but the vertical tarsal blood vessels are visible.

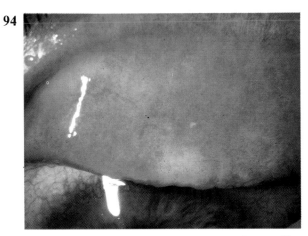

94 **Atopic conjunctivitis**. There are many fine papillae present in the everted upper tarsal plate. Hyperaemia and cellular infiltration disguise the anatomical structure of the normal tarsal blood vessels.

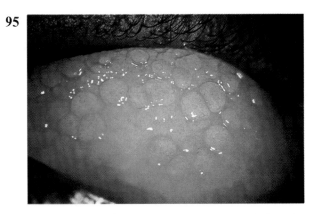

95 **Vernal catarrh**. The everted upper tarsal plate demonstrates cobblestone papillae. The disease is not active, and the condition is not necessarily symptomatic, as the papillae themselves do not cause symtoms.

THE EYE IN HAY FEVER AND VERNAL CATARRH

Hay fever conjunctivitis is a common component of hay fever, and the ocular signs can usually be managed without ophthalmological referral. The condition is episodic, and the eyes appear normal between episodes. When signs are present, they consist merely of hyperaemia and slight swelling of the tarsal conjunctiva, and some chemosis of the bulbar conjunctiva. There are no long-term consequences.

Vernal catarrh is more serious and long-lasting. The condition is commonest in children between five and 15 years of age, and it usually remits in adult life. The typical patient has multiple positive skin-prick tests to a broad range of allergens. The symptoms of vernal catarrh are much more severe than those of hay fever conjunctivitis. Itching is a major symptom, together with a copious discharge of lardaceous mucopurulent material. Photophobia can be extremely severe on waking in the morning, and children may often require periods of 30-45 minutes for adaptation to daylight. The signs of vernal catarrh are of large cobblestone papillae, and of mucopurulent discharge in the conjunctival sac. The active disease may be associated with the formation of microerosions in the upper half of the cornea, and this sign indicates a need for urgent treatment. Severe vernal catarrh can lead to chronic corneal ulceration, and can thus be a threat to sight. Referral to an ophthalmologist is required in these circumstances.

Atopic conjunctivitis is often seen in atopic adults. The appearances in the tarsal plates are different to those seen in vernal catarrh in children, in that the papillae are fine and closely packed together, producing a hyperaemic 'felty' appearance of the upper tarsal plate, which disguises the usual anatomy of the vascular arcade. The symptoms are itching and a chronic discharge, and there may be a chronic keratitis. In some adult patients, severe herpetic keratitis can be a complicating problem.

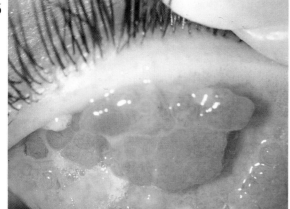

96 Active vernal catarrh, with large papillae on the everted upper tarsal plate. There is a copious discharge of mucopurulent material, associated with severe itching and photophobia.

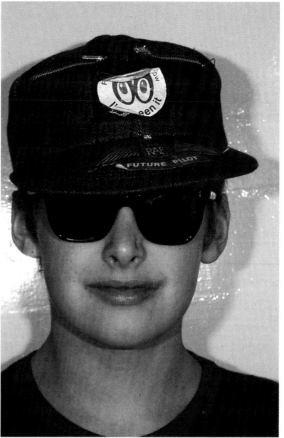

97 Severe vernal catarrh often induces severe photophobia, as shown by the appearance of this typical patient.

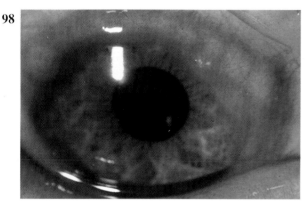

98 Limbal vernal catarrh. This type of vernal catarrh is most commonly found in the Middle East and Third World countries. The papillae are found on the conjunctiva and they encroach onto the limbus, and are associated with infiltrations of inflammatory cells (Tranter spots). In this type of vernal disease, the changes in the tarsal plates are much less marked.

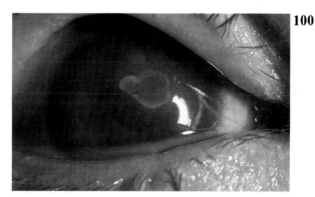

100 Chronic corneal ulcer in vernal catarrh. The ulcer is stained with fluorescein. This condition is associated with severe, handicapping symptoms. The ulcers are generally oval, with the horizontal diameter the longest. They result from the recurrent deposition of sticky mucus, which prevents the re-establishment of the epithelial layer. Operative removal of the plaque results in rapid regeneration of the epithelium.

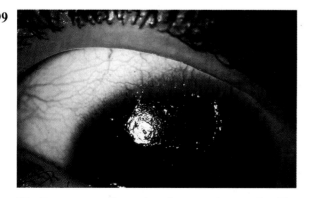

99 Large corneal erosion in vernal catarrh. The erosion is seen in the upper part of the cornea, and it results from the coalescence of many microerosions. It is on epithelial deficits such as this that the deposition of sticky mucus may lead to chronic and persistent ulceration.

101

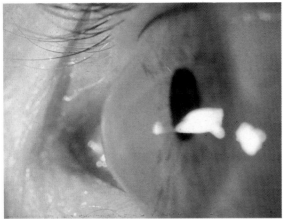

102

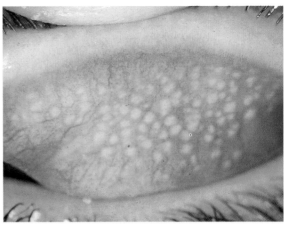

101 Keratoconus in an atopic patient. In this condition there is central filling of the cornea, associated with a steepening of the corneal curvature. It is associated with considerable visual deterioration, and can be initially treated with a contact lens, but where the thinning becomes associated with corneal scarring, and where contact lenses can no longer be tolerated, a corneal graft can be performed. Keratoconus is found in association with eczema and asthma or hay fever in approximately 50 per cent of patients. It may also be seen in patients with vernal catarrh.

102 Contact lens allergy. Contact lenses can induce allergic responses in the upper tarsal plate similar to those seen in vernal catarrh. The papillae, however, have white apices and are not so large, even though the condition is known by ophthalmologists as giant papillary conjunctivitis (GPC). Symptoms and clinical signs are not always obvious, but contact lens intolerance due to this cause is becoming more common. It usually responds to a change in contact lens material.

103

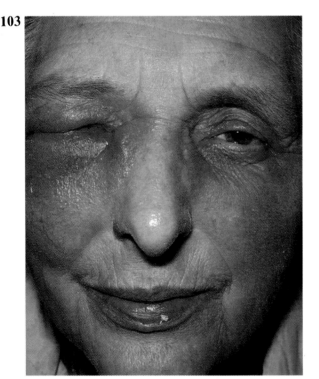

104

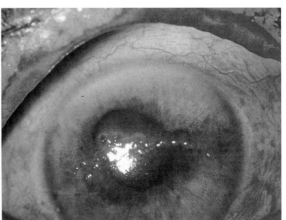

103 Allergy to eye drops. This woman developed a bilateral delayed hypersensitivity response in her eyelids and cheeks following the administration of eye drops. Atropine and neomycin are the two common causes.

104 The dry eye. This may occur in isolation or association with sarcoidosis or the connective tissue disorders. The cornea and conjunctiva are stained with Rose Bengal drops which highlight many microerosions on the ocular surface. There is also adherent mucus on the corneal surface producing mucus plaque keratitis.

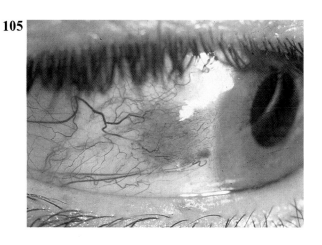

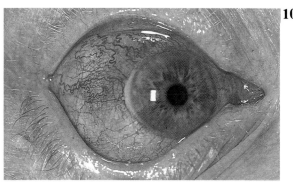

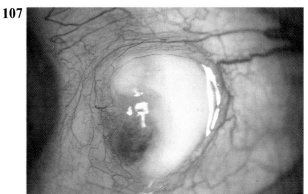

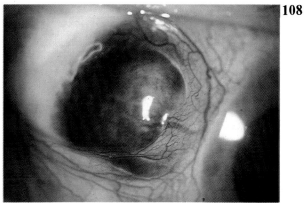

107 Scleromalacia perforans occurring in a male patient with severe rheumatoid arthritis. The condition is associated with inflammation in the conjunctiva and sclera surrounding it, and it responds poorly to topical and systemic therapy. In this patient treatment with immunosuppressive therapy eventually resulted in a therapeutic response.

108 Necrotising scleritis in a patient with circulating immune complexes suffering from Wegener's granulomatosis. The condition ultimately responded to cyclophosphamide, and the inflammation slowly resolved.

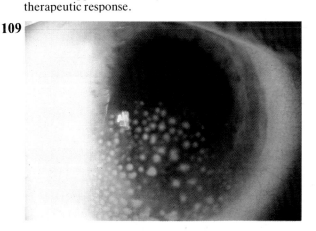

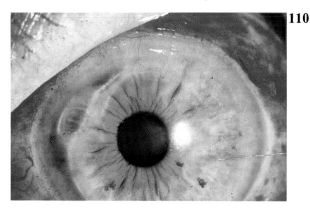

109 Uveitis. Keratitic precipitates demonstrated by a 'scleral scatter' technique of illumination with a slit lamp, showing large 'mutton fat' deposits. The cause of the uveitis was unknown in this case.

110 The peripheral corneal melting syndrome is occasionally associated with connective tissue disorders including rheumatoid arthritis, polyarteritis nodosa and Wegener's granulomatosis. Its mechanism is unknown. There is peripheral thinning of the cornea with minimal vascularisation and the condition poses a serious threat to vision.

111

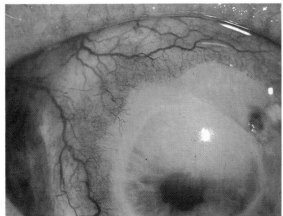

111 Peripheral keratitis with thinning in association with necrotising scleritis (see **108**), in a patient with severe rheumatoid arthritis.

112

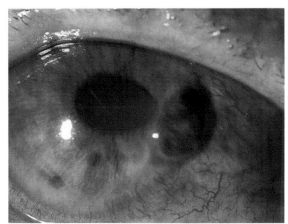

112 Perforated cornea with prolapsed iris may be the end result of the peripheral corneal melting syndrome, as in this patient with severe rheumatoid arthritis.

113

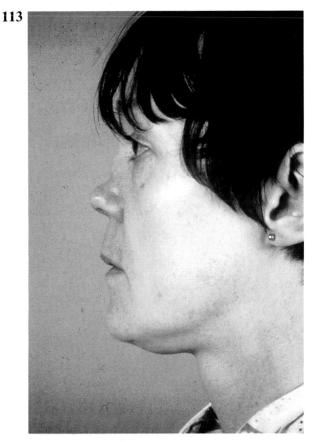

113 Wegener's granulomatosis is seen in association with the peripheral corneal melting syndrome. This patient also shows the characteristic collapsed nasal septum associated with the disease. Her Wegener's granulomatosis responded to treatment with cyclophosphamide, but the peripheral corneal melting syndrome required a combination of corticosteroids and azathioprine.

114

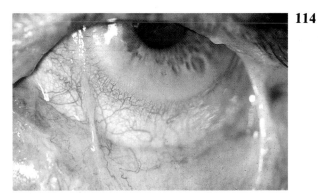

114 Cicatricial mucous membrane pemphigoid, showing shrinkage of the conjunctiva, manifest as folds when the lower lid is pulled downwards.

115

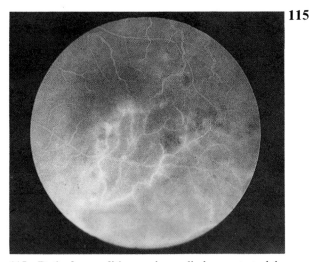

115 Retinal vasculitis can be well demonstrated by fluorescein angiography. It may be associated with the immune complex diseases, and may present as retinal haemorrhages and exudates with intraretinal oedema. Occasionally haemorrhages may spread into the vitreous, and this may cause visual disability.

STEROIDS AND THE EYE

Topical corticosteroids are of use in many of the inflammatory diseases of the eye caused by allergic and chronic infective disease, but their long-term use can be damaging, as cataract and glaucoma can occur, leading to permanent loss of sight. Even in the short-term, they reduce the defences of the eye against infection, and can result in very severe herpetic disease where the diagnosis has not been accurately made. Topical corticosteroid treatment should always be monitored by an ophthalmologist.

HERPES SIMPLEX AND THE EYE

Herpes simplex infection is a relatively common and dangerous complication of allergic eye disease. Atopic individuals seem prone to herpes infections of the eye in any case, and steroid therapy is often an important additional factor.

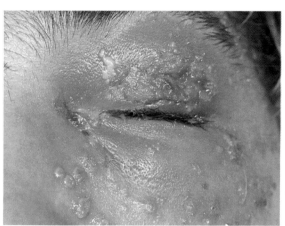

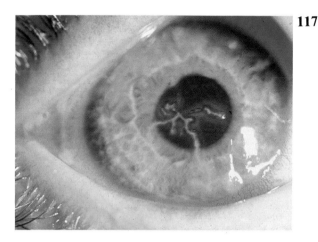

116   Primary herpes simplex virus infection around the eye, occurring in a highly atopic individual. It is often such subjects who get a particularly severe viral disease of this nature, and it is not uncommon for the eyes to become involved with disease recurrence.

117   A primary dendritic ulcer stained with fluorescein dye. The ulcer is due to herpes simplex virus proliferation in the epithelial layer of the cornea. Dendritic ulcers can be treated with antiviral drops or ointments such as vidarabine and acyclovir, and treatment should be initiated as soon as the diagnosis is made, but the patient should also be referred to an ophthalmologist.

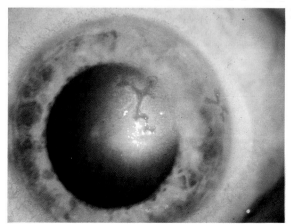

118   Two recurrent dendrites occurring over an area of stromal infiltration. Stromal opacification may occur as a result of the inappropriate use of topical corticosteroid in this condition.

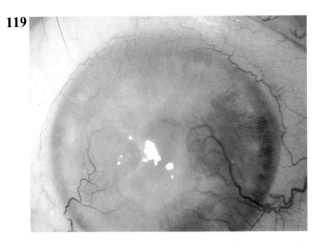

119 Diffuse stromal keratitis associated with corneal vascularisation. The cause is herpes simplex virus invasion of the deeper corneal tissue, and severe disease of this kind can occur when topical corticosteroids are erroneously employed for the treatment of dendritic ulcers. Corneal opacity of this type is one of the most common indications for corneal grafting in the developed world.

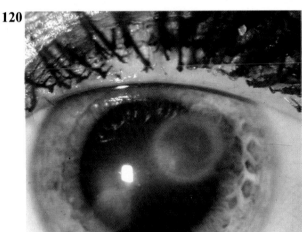

120 An immune ring due to the herpes simplex virus in the stroma. This fascinating appearance mimics that normally seen when radial immunodiffusion is carried out on agar gel, and the ring results from the precipitation of immune complexes.

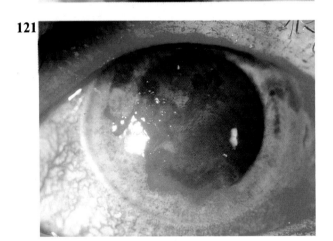

121 A geographic ulcer due to herpes simplex virus, demonstrated with Rose Bengal drops. The patient had been treated inappropriately with topical corticosteroid drops.

6 ALLERGY IN THE NOSE AND EAR

RHINITIS

Seasonal rhinitis is the commonest of all allergic diseases. Up to 20 per cent of the population of western countries suffer from non-viral rhinitis, and about 50 per cent of cases are allergic in origin. Allergic rhinitis may be *seasonal* or *perennial*.

The commonest cause of *seasonal* rhinitis is pollen allergy. In the UK grass pollens are the commonest allergens, the most important being timothy and rye grass. In North America, allergy to ragweed pollen is a common cause, while in some parts of the Middle East prosoba tree pollen is important. Moulds are another cause of seasonal symptoms. The range of allergens in the air varies from time to time and from place to place (e.g. see **22**). Seasonal rhinitis is often accompanied by conjunctivitis, and sometimes by asthma or urticaria.

Perennial rhinitis is most commonly caused by allergy to the faeces of the house dust mite (see **23**), though the symptoms may show seasonal exacerbation, being worst during the winter when the mite population is greatest. Allergy to cats, dogs, horses and other domestic animals may also cause perennial rhinitis, while occasional exposure may cause intermittent symptoms.

Patients with *allergic rhinitis* have positive skin tests and sometimes also an elevated serum IgE level. Patients with similar symptoms who have negative skin tests and a normal serum IgE are said to have *nonspecific rhinitis*. It is probable that some of these patients have a reaction to an unidentified allergen, and that others have an allergic reaction confined to the nose—a possibility which is supported by the presence of eosinophils in nasal secretions or blood (non-allergic rhinitis with eosinophilia syndrome—NARES)

Vasomotor rhinitis is a non-allergic condition characterised by hyper-responsiveness of the nasal mucosa to stimuli such as smoke, temperature changes, alcohol and emotion. It can be difficult to distinguish clinically from allergic rhinitis, and a degree of vasomotor instability often accompanies severe nasal allergy, so that the nose becomes hyper-reactive to irritants as well as allergens.

Table 26.   A classification of rhinitis

Allergic	Seasonal
	Perennial
	Perennial with seasonal variation
Chronic nonspecific	Without eosinophilia
	With eosinophilia (NARES)
Vasomotor	Primary
	Secondary
Salicylate-associated rhinitis with nasal polyps	
Infectious	Viral
	Bacterial
Rhinitis medicamentosa	Nasal decongestant sprays
	Other drugs
Other rarer causes	Metabolic
	Neoplastic
	Foreign body
	CSF rhinorrhoea

Table 27. Clinical and laboratory features of four common types of rhinitis

	Allergic rhinitis	Nonspecific rhinitis	Vasomotor rhinitis	Salicylate associated rhinitis
Age of onset	Child or adult	Adult	Adult	Adult
Congestion/Rhinorrhoea	++	++	++	+++
Sneezing/Itching	+++	+	−	−
Nasal mucosa appearance	Variable	Variable	Variable	Variable
Nasal polyps	Uncommon	Uncommon	Rare	Common
Skin tests	+++	−	−	−
Eosinophilia	++	++	−	++
High plasma IgE	+/−	−	−	−

122

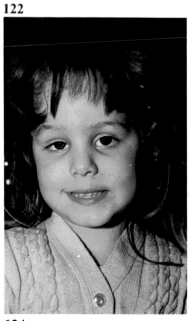

123

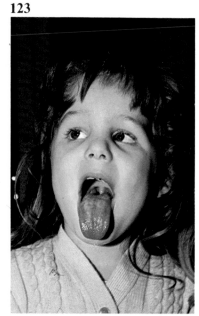

122 to 125 The characteristic facial appearance of a child with nasal allergy. This 5-year-old girl has infraorbital oedema and a characteristic gaping appearance of the mouth, through which she normally breathes as a result of nasal obstruction. Her large, fleshy tonsils can be seen clearly, and similarly enlarged adenoids make a major contribution to the nasal obstruction. She also has chronic rhinitis, as shown by her habit of rubbing her nose to relieve itching, and by the characteristic 'allergic salute', in which the fingers and palm of the hand are rubbed upwards over the tip of the nose.

124

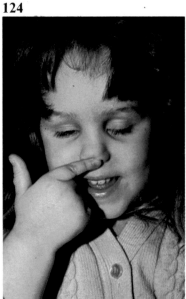

125

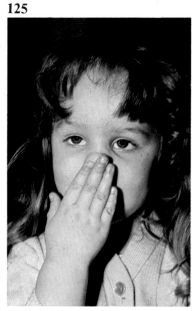

126 The peak nasal inspiratory flow meter. Nasal obstruction is a prominent feature of most allergic disorders of the nose, but subjective sensations are not a reliable guide to nasal patency, and an objective measure of obstruction should be helpful in the assessment of obstruction and its response to therapy. Many devices to measure nasal airway resistance have been described, but most require laboratory equipment and none has proved as reliable as peak flow measurements are in asthma (see **159-166**).

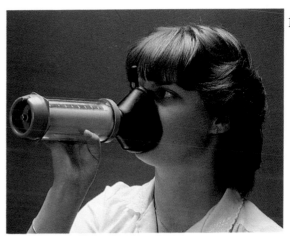

Shown here is one of the more encouraging recent developments in the field, a simple handheld device which is adapted from the low-reading version of the Wright mini peak flow meter (**160**). This peak nasal inspiratory flow meter has been found useful in nasal provocation testing with allergens, in the home monitoring of nasal airway function, in assessing response to medical treatment, and in assessing the need for and response to nasal surgery. It has the advantage of being relatively cheap and portable, and its reproducibility and sensitivity corresponds reasonably well with more complicated methods such as rhinomanometry.

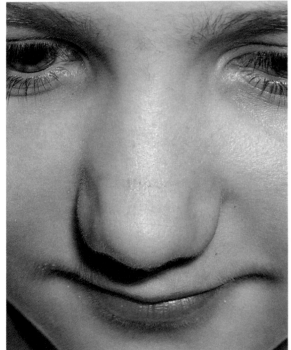

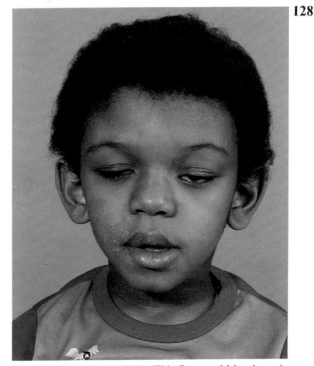

127 The pigmented nasal crease which results from a chronic allergic salute. It is seen here in a 10-year-old girl with perennial rhinitis. The shape of her nose suggests possible internal obstruction by polyps, but none were found.

128 Another atopic child. This 7-year-old boy's main problem was asthma, but he has characteristic allergic facies, with a lethargic expression, infraorbital and peri-oral oedema, early Dennie Morgan infraorbital folds (see **28**), a swollen and congested nose and some facial eczema, especially around the mouth.

129

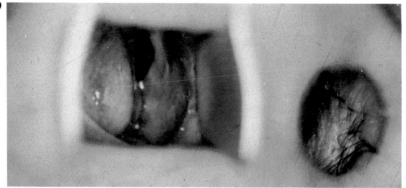

130

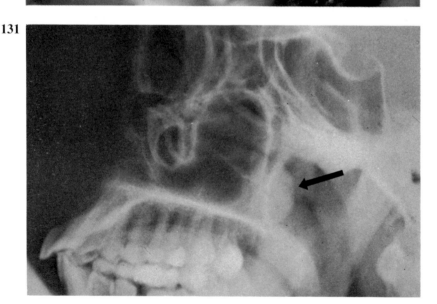

131

129 Acute rhinitis in seasonal allergy. The nasal mucous membrane is oedematous, so the inferior turbinate abuts against the septum, causing obstruction. A similar appearance is seen in perennial rhinitis and in the common cold, though the infected mucous membrane tends to be redder than that in allergy. In allergic rhinitis increased mucus production leads to a 'runny nose', but persistent purulent discharge usually implies co-existent sinusitis (see **134**).

130 Chronic rhinitis resulting from long-term, uncontrolled house dust mite allergy. The patient complained of a persistent but variable nasal obstruction and of a postnasal discharge of mucus. Nasal steroid or sodium cromoglycate treatment often improves symptoms in chronic allergic rhinitis, and they may also be helped by oral antihistamines and by other measures such as antigen avoidance or desensitisation to the dust mite faecal antigen. Sometimes minor surgery on the nasal turbinates is necessary to reduce the nasal obstruction. Vasoconstrictor drops or sprays should not be used—indeed, their chronic use is a *cause* of chronic rhinitis (rhinitis medicamentosa).

131 Enlarged inferior turbinates in chronic allergic rhinitis. These may be seen with a post-nasal mirror; if so, they often look like mulberries and may be termed 'mulberry ends'. If not, they can be demonstrated on xray. The posterior ends of the enlarged turbinates produce a large polypoidal mass obstructing the posterior choanae (arrowed). Clinically, they may be difficult to distinguish from nasal polyps. Removal of the posterior ends of the turbinates often relieves symptoms.

132 Enlarged adenoids. The post-nasal space is often very difficult to see in a child, but a lateral xray may show the airway to be almost completely occluded by a large adenoidal pad, as here (arrowed). Adenoidal enlargement is common in both atopic and non-atopic children, but it may compound the problem of nasal obstruction in children with allergic rhinitis.

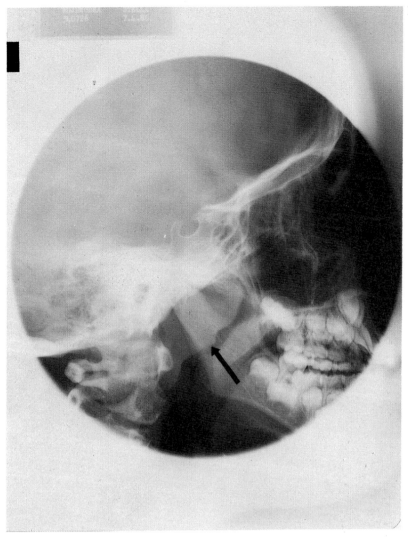

133 Adenoids following operative removal. The adenoids usually regress before puberty and their operative removal should usually be avoided if possible. Sometimes, though, removal is indicated when there are marked nasal and aural symptoms—as present here.

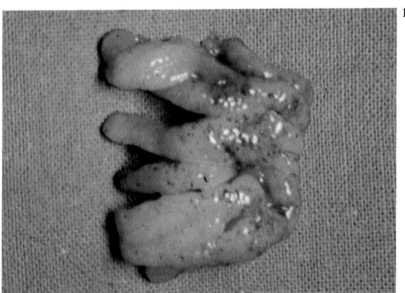

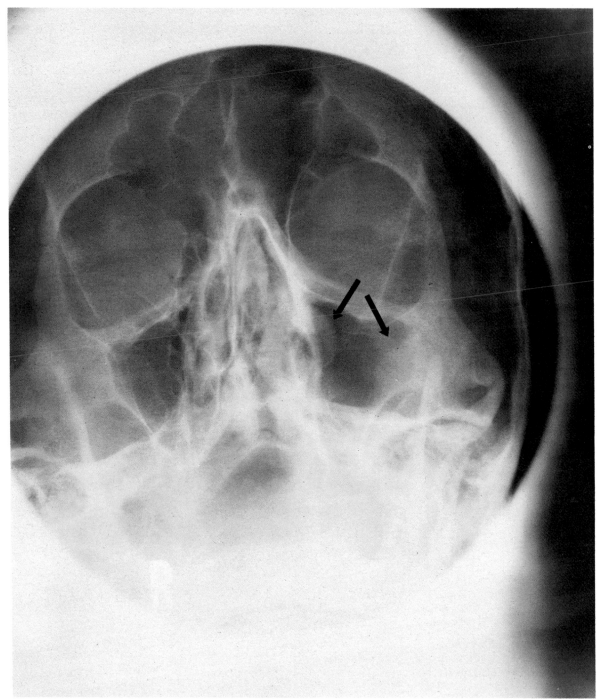

134 Sinusitis, with mucosal polyps (arrowed) on the lateral and medial walls of the left maxillary antrum. Seen here in a 30-year-old man with hay fever. Sinusitis is usually the result of infection rather than a direct manifestation of allergy, but infection is undoubtedly encouraged by congestion of the nasal mucosa, which may prevent normal drainage of the maxillary antra.

NASAL POLYPS

Nasal polyps are rare in vasomotor rhinitis and uncommon in both allergic and non-specific rhinitis, but they are characteristic of 'salicylate-associated rhinitis'. This syndrome usually consists of the triad of rhinitis with nasal polyps, sinusitis and asthma, and all three conditions are exacerbated by aspirin and other non-steroidal anti-inflammatory drugs (and by salicylate-rich foods). The mechanism of this type of rhinitis is not fully understood. It is usually associated with eosinophilia, but the serum IgE level is normal, and skin tests are usually negative. A non-allergic mechanism is likely.

Nasal polyps may cause unremitting nasal obstruction and anosmia. Surgical excision may be required, but the polyps often respond well to local or systemic corticosteroid treatment, though this may need to be continued indefinitely to prevent recurrence.

Nasal polyps most commonly originate in the ethmoidal air cells and grow into the nose from under the middle turbinate. 'Antro-choanal polyps' originate in the maxillary antrum and prolapse into the nose via the hiatus semilunaris. They are commonly unilateral, and they may reach a considerable length, hanging down into the nasopharynx.

Polyps are benign, but it is important to exclude tumours in the differential diagnosis, especially where a polyp is unilateral, and avulsed polyps should always be examined microscopically.

Caution: In children it is essential to consider the possibility of a meningocoele, which may resemble a nasal polyp—avulsion of a meningocoele is a catastrophic error.

135

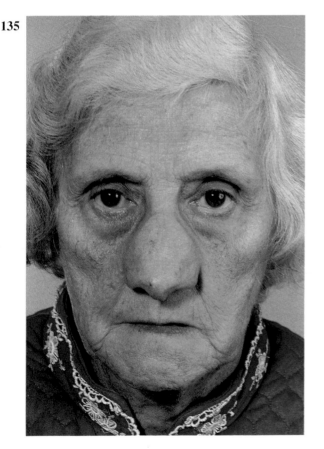

135 Nasal polyps. This 74-year-old woman complained of near-total nasal obstruction and anosmia. Her nose was obviously enlarged.

136

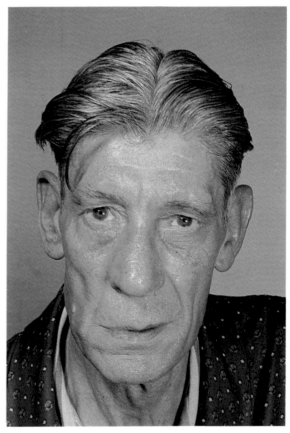

136 Nasal polyps. A 62-year-old man with a similar appearance. He also had sinusitis and aspirin-provoked asthma.

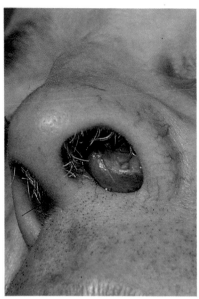 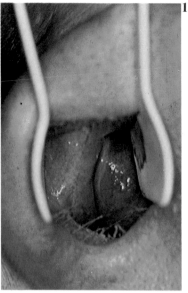 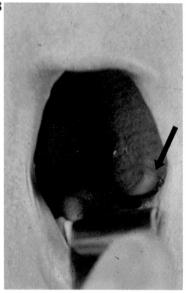

137 and 138 Large nasal polyps. These are often easily seen without special instruments, though a better view can usually be obtained through a nasal speculum or a large otoscope.

139 Polyp in the oropharynx. Large posterior polyps may extend below the soft palate and present in the oropharynx (arrowed). A unilateral polyp of this kind is usually an antrochoanal polyp.

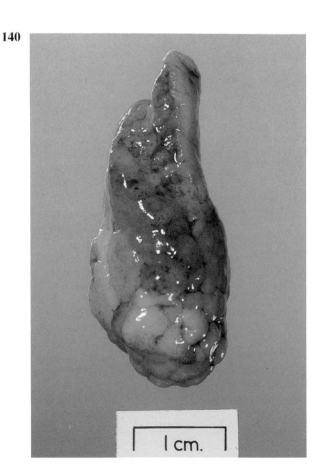

140 Nasal polyp removed from a 42-year-old woman with asthma and aspirin sensitivity. This polyp is about 3 cm long, but many polyps are larger when they are removed, especially if they originate in the mucosa of the maxillary antrum, and a length of 6 to 10 cm is not unusual.

ALLERGY AND THE EAR

The skin of the auricle and the external auditory meatus may be affected by the same allergic disorders as the skin elsewhere. Two especially common examples of contact dermatitis are nickel sensitivity from ear-rings (see **46**) and sensitivity to antimicrobial or other drugs used in ear drops. The ear moulds used in hearing aids may also cause contact reactions, though these are unlikely when hypo-allergenic or gold-plated moulds are used.

141

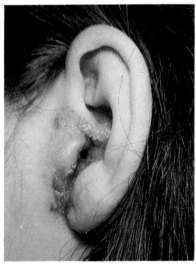

142

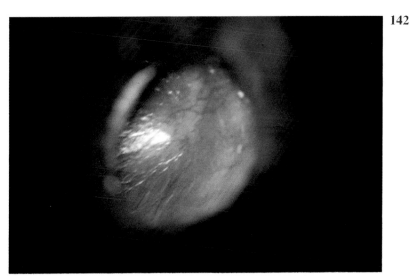

141 Otitis externa with sensitivity to ear drops. This woman had a mild otitis externa which became much more severe after treatment with chloramphenicol ear drops. Contact sensitivity to chloramphenicol is quite common, and a similar reaction may result from the use of drops containing neomycin (as in the eye—see **103**).

142 Secretory otitis media with minimal change in the drum. The tympanic membrane is slightly brownish in colour and a little hyperaemic, but could well be taken for a normal drum. Nevertheless, this child had a significant hearing impairment and a tenacious middle-ear exudate.

143 Secretory otitis media with marked changes in the drum. The diagnosis is obvious here. The tympanic membrane is retracted, the malleus is prominent, and parts of the drum have a characteristic golden colour.

143

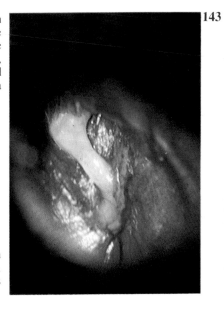

144

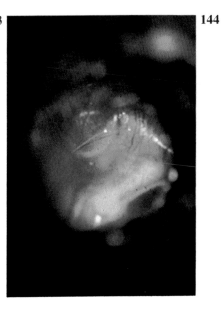

144 Bubbles and a fluid level in the middle ear may be seen in partially resolved secretory otitis media.

In the inner ear, allergy has been considered as a cause of Ménière's disease but careful studies have failed to show any evidence for this. A link with autoimmunity has recently been suggested, but more research is required in this field. Other work is looking at a possible role of allergy in sudden hearing loss.

In the middle ear, there may be an association between atopy and secretory otitis media (SOM), a disorder of childhood characterised by hearing loss and a chronic viscid effusion in the middle ear—'glue ear'. Both recurrent acute otitis media and SOM seem to be encouraged by blockage of the Eustachian tubes, and it is likely that this blockage can be provoked by the congestion associated with allergic rhinitis, in the same way that allergic rhinitis may provoke sinusitis, as well as by enlarged adenoids (see **132**). However, there is no evidence that allergy has any direct role in the changes within the ear, and certainly no evidence to support the suggestion that allergy to milk or foods may be a directly causative factor.

SOM is least common in the summer months, when allergic rhinitis is commonest, and antihistamines and vasoconstrictors have no significant effect on the condition. SOM may occur in both atopic and non-atopic children, and there is no evidence of a greater incidence in the former group. Both SOM and atopic allergy are common in childhood, and a very large study involving both skin-prick testing and tympanometry would be required to clarify their relationship.

The treatment of chronic serous otitis media (CSOM) often involves the insertion of a grommet to ventilate the middle ear cleft, and treatment is the same whether or not the child has evidence of atopy. The condition rarely persists beyond 11 years of age, so treatment should be conservative whenever possible, but 'glue ear' has potentially serious educational and other consequences (**145**) and should not be ignored.

145

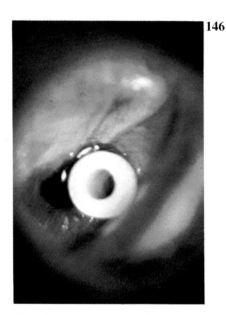

145 Grossly altered drum in chronic serous otitis media. The lower arrow points to the indrawn drum; the upper arrow shows the incudo-stapedial joint. CSOM may persist for decades if undiagnosed, and can be a cause of longstanding deafness.

146

146 A grommet inserted in the tympanic membrane to ventilate the middle ear is the most effective treatment for CSOM, though it is not required in all cases. It acts as a substitute for the Eustachian tube, and hearing and the appearance of the drum usually return to normal. The grommet is usually extruded within 6 to 12 months, and it may need to be replaced if CSOM recurs. Some modern grommets are designed to stay in the drum for more prolonged periods.

7 ALLERGIC CONDITIONS OF THE LUNGS

Allergic reactions play a part in a number of lung disorders. As elsewhere in the body, the classification into types I to IV can be helpful (see Chapter 1), but many disorders involve more than one immune mechanism. Thus extrinsic allergic alveolitis, bronchopulmonary aspergillosis and the Churg-Strauss syndrome probably involve interactions between mechanisms of types I, III, and IV, while Wegener's granulomatosis and sarcoidosis involve types III and IV. Even in bronchial asthma—often considered a classical type I reaction—other mechanisms are undoubtedly involved.

Table 28. Mechanisms of immunological lung injury

Immune type	I	II	III	IV
Alternative name	Immediate hypersensitivity	Cytotoxic antibody	Antigen-antibody immune complex	Delayed-type cell-mediated
Cells involved	B Mast cell Basophil Eosinophil	B or K Macrophage	B Polymorph Platelet	T Macrophage Giant and epithelioid
Immunoglobulin	IgE	IgE; IgM	IgG	-
Clinical disorder				
Respiratory	Asthma Rhinitis	Goodpasture's syndrome	Sarcoidosis Rheumatoid lung Rheumato- pneumoconiosis Fibrosing alveolitis	Sarcoidosis Nitrofurantoin lung Allergic alveolitis Bronchopulmonary aspergillosis Wegener's granulomatosis
Systemic	Conjunctivitis Urticaria Angioedema Atopic eczema	Glomerulonephritis	Serum sickness Systemic lupus erythematosus Behcêt's syndrome	Graft rejection Contact dermatitis Churg-Strauss syndrome
Appropriate immunological investigations	Immediate skin tests Serum IgE RAST	Alveolar and glomerular immuno-fluorescence	Circulating immune complexes Complement conversion High ESR Immunofluorescence	Skin patch tests Lymphocyte transformation Macrophage-migration inhibition Cell-mediated cytotoxicity

ASTHMA

Asthma is commonly defined as: 'a disorder of function characterised by dyspnoea caused by widespread narrowing of peripheral airways in the lungs, varying in severity over short periods of time either spontaneously or with treatment'.

Asthma is a common disorder. Its prevalence is highest in the second decade of life, when it may affect 10-15 per cent of the population in developed countries such as the UK, the USA and New Zealand. It is much less common in most

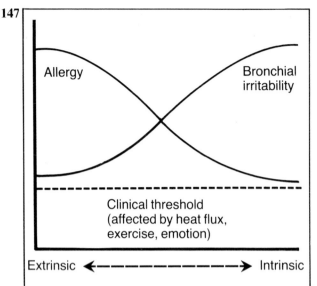

147 Contributory factors in asthma.

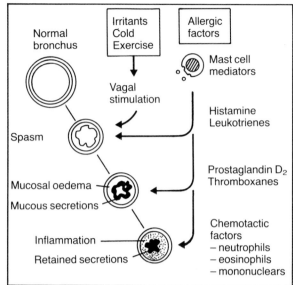

148 The pathogenesis of asthma. A schematic representation of the current understanding of probable pathogenic mechanisms.

Table 29. Common provoking factors in asthma

- Inhaled environmental allergens
- Occupational allergens
- Atmospheric pollution
- Irritant dusts, smoke and fumes
- Occupational irritants
- Cold air
- Exercise
- Emotion
- Aspirin and other non-steroidal anti-inflammatory drugs
- Beta-blocking drugs
- Foods

Asian countries. Occupational asthma is a common problem in those exposed to sensitizing substances in industry.

In non-occupational asthma the allergens involved are similar to those causing allergic rhinitis and conjunctivitis, though pollen is a less common cause of asthma (perhaps because of the relatively large size of pollen grains) and dust mite faecal particles are probably the commonest cause of allergic asthma worldwide.

Asthma is accompanied by bronchial hyper-activity—an increased responsiveness of the airways to non-specific stimuli. Although the degree of hyperreactivity may be influenced by allergic mechanisms, its pathogenesis is unclear, and non-allergic factors are also involved. There is much support for the view that established asthma is an inflammatory condition.

Occupational asthma

Well over 200 different causes of occupational asthma have been recognised, and seven of these are recognised for statutory compensation purposes in the UK. Some occupational materials produce asthma by a classic Type I mechanism, and specific IgE antibody can be found in the serum. In other cases, the mechanism is still unknown.

Table 30. The seven most important causes of occupational asthma in the UK

IgE related

Allergens from animals (including insects)	Laboratories
Allergens from flour and grain	Farmers, millers, grain handlers
Proteolytic enzymes	Manufacture of 'biological' washing powders (but not their use)
Complex salts of platinum	Metal refining
Acid anhydrides and polyamine hardening agents	Industrial coatings

Non-IgE related

Isocyanates	Polyurethane varnishes, industrial coatings
Colophony fumes	Soldering, electronics industry

Classification of asthma

Asthma is often divided into two sub-groups:

- Extrinsic asthma—a definite external cause is implied
- Intrinsic or cryptogenic asthma—where no causative agent can be identified.

Those with extrinsic asthma are typically atopic individuals who show positive skin-prick reactions to common inhaled allergens, whereas those with intrinsic asthma are not. Ninety per cent of asthmatic children have positive skin tests to one or more substances in the standard battery (see Table 5) whereas only 50 per cent of adults do.

The extrinsic/intrinsic classification is of little practical value. Non-atopic patients may develop asthma in middle age from extrinsic causes such as sensitization to occupational agents, intolerance to aspirin, or the use of beta-blockers for the treatment of hypertension or angina. Extrinsic causes should thus be considered in all cases of asthma and avoided whenever possible. Other treatment for the two sub-groups is similar.

Table 31.   Physical signs in asthma

In the acute attack
- Tachypnoea
- Hyperinflated chest, with symmetrically reduced chest wall movement
- Prolonged expiration with vesicular breath sounds
- Expiratory wheeze
- Cough—especially in children
- Thick yellow-green sputum—does not necessarily indicate infection
- No mediastinal displacement
- Normal percussion
- Normal vocal resonance

In the severe acute attack
- Tachycardia
- The wheeze may disappear as a result of reduced air-flow
- Variable jugular venous pressure (high during expiration)
- Pulsus paradoxus (an exaggerated fall in systolic BP on inspiration)
- Rapid progress to life-threatening respiratory distress with cyanosis

In chronic or recurrent episodic asthma
- Signs of other allergic disorder may be present
- Pigeon chest—if asthma started in childhood
- Growth retardation—if asthma started in childhood
- Cushingoid features if long-term systemic steroid treatment used

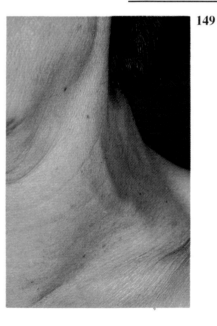

149 **150**

149 and 150   The jugular venous pulsation in severe acute asthma. The great respiratory effort in severe acute asthma results in large intrathoracic pressure swings. These lead in turn to variations in the venous pressure. The jugular venous pressure is high during expiration with filling of the neck veins (**149**). On inspiration the neck veins empty (**150**).

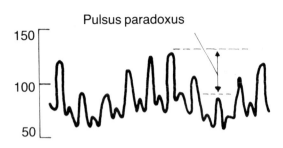

Pulsus paradoxus

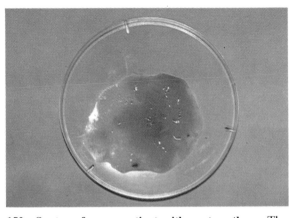

151 Pulsus paradoxus in acute asthma. The arterial pressure trace shows a variation in pressure of 30 mmHg between inspiration and expiration. Pulsus paradoxus is defined as more than a 10 per cent or 10 mmHg fall in systolic pressure with inspiration. It is an exaggeration of the normal finding of decreased arterial pressure with inspiration. The sign is not diagnostic of asthma, as it is also found in severe fixed air-flow obstruction.

152 Sputum from a patient with acute asthma. The sputum is thick and gelatinous, and may often be yellow or green. This colouring reflects the large number of eosinophils and other cell debris within the sputum, and does not necessarily indicate infection. Microscopic examination of a smear of sputum in asthma commonly shows sputum eosinophilia (see **16**).

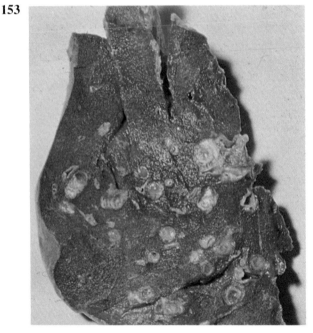

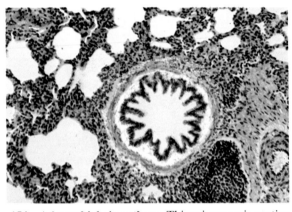

154 A bronchiole in asthma. This microscopic section shows narrowing of the lumen caused by constriction of smooth muscle. Lung tissue from asthmatics shows hypertrophy of smooth muscle in the bronchial walls, thickening of the mucosa, hypertrophy of the mucus glands and eosinophilic infiltration. Mucus plugs may block the airways.

153 Asthma still kills, as shown by this post-mortem lung. Plugs of viscid mucus project from the lumen of the sectioned bronchi. Despite apparently improved management, the death rate from asthma has remained similar over the past 20-30 years.

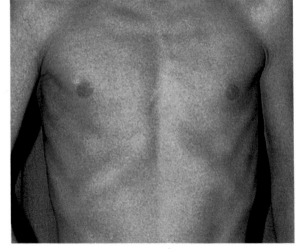

155 Hyperinflated chest in chronic asthma. This 10-year-old child suffered growth retardation. The chest is hyperinflated and the lower ribs and costal margin splayed out. The deformity is called Harrison's sulcus.

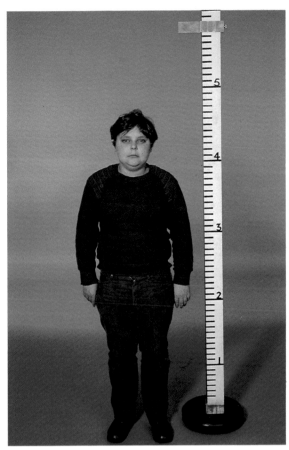

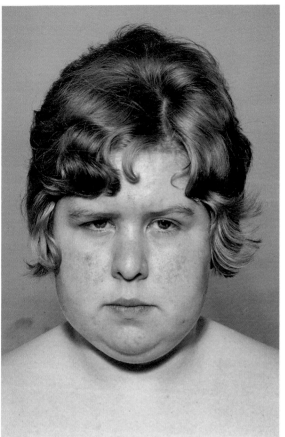

156 Severe growth retardation in a 17-year-old boy with chronic asthma. As the scale shows, he is 4′8″ tall. Asthma itself causes growth retardation, but here—as so often—chronic systemic steroid treatment has compounded the problem. Fortunately inhaled steroids do not have the same growth-retarding effect as systemic steroids, but systemic treatment is still required in some patients. Whenever possible, steroid treatment should be administered in short-term 'pulses' or on an alternate-day basis, as these manoeuvres may help to prevent unwanted side-effects.

157 Cushingoid facial features and buffalo hump. Seen here in a 15-year-old girl with chronic asthma who had been receiving long-term oral prednisolone therapy. This picture dates from 1966, and such extreme cases are fortunately uncommon now.

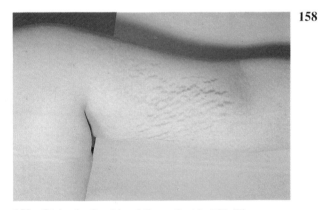

158 Striae in the skin of the patient in 157. These were also the result of long-term systemic steroid therapy.

Investigations in asthma

Respiratory function tests are both an important initial investigation in asthma and a valuable guide to its progress and treatment.

The simplest and most useful measurements are:

● The forced expiratory volume in one second (FEV$_1$), the forced vital capacity (FVC) and their ratio (FEV$_1$/FVC).

● The peak expiratory flow rate (PEFR).

Measurement of the FEV$_1$ and FVC requires a spirometer, but cheaper and simpler devices are available to measure PEFR, and these may be used at home by the patient.

159 Peak flow meter in use. The patient takes in a deep breath, and then makes a maximal expiratory effort through the instrument. It is usual to repeat the procedure three times and to record the highest PEFR reading obtained. This can then be compared with a nomogram which allows for the patient's sex, age and weight (see **161** and **162**), and plotted on a chart to show progress or response to treatment.

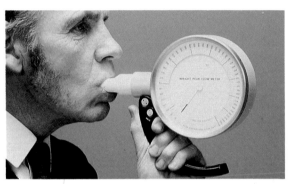

159

160 Mini peak flow meter in use. This device produces similar results to the meter shown in **159**, but it is less expensive and thus more suitable for home use by individual patients.

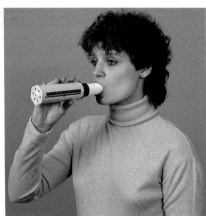

160

161

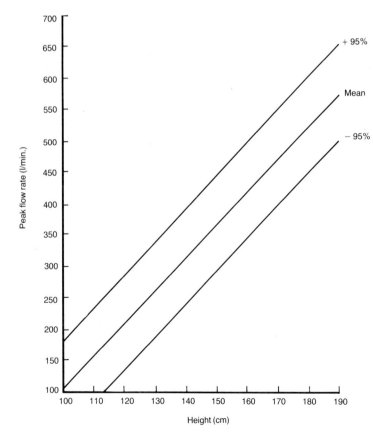

161 Peak expiratory flow rate in normal children. This nomogram is based upon data from Godfrey, S., et al, *British Journal of Diseases of the Chest, 1970,* **64**, 15. Three hundred and eighty two normal boys and girls aged 5–18 were tested, and each child blew five times into a standard Wright Peak Flow Meter, with the highest reading being accepted in each case. The outer lines of the nomogram indicate that the results of 95 per cent of the children fell within these boundaries.

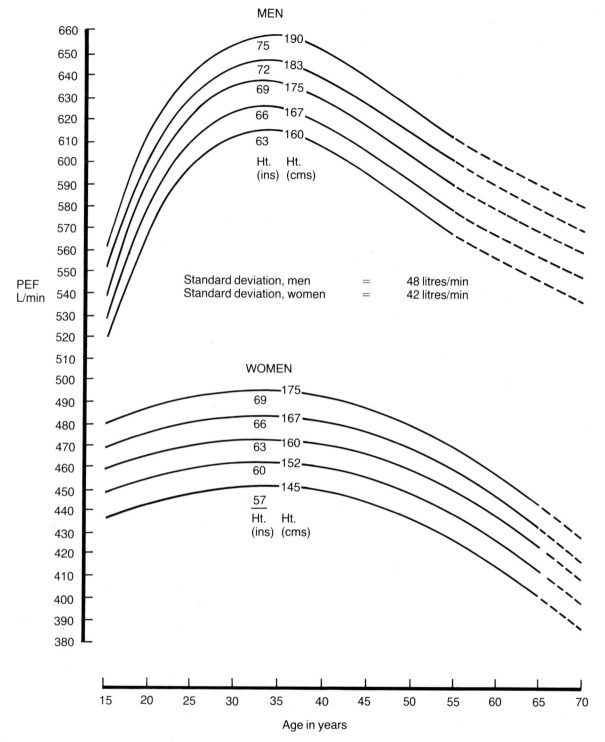

162 Peak expiratory flow rate in normal adult subjects. Observed values can be simply compared with normal values on this chart. In general, values of PEFR up to 100 l/m less than predicted in men, and up to 85 l/m less than predicted in women, can be considered to be within normal limits.

A series of readings over a period of time have more value than a single reading, and response to an inhaled bronchodilator drug can give a useful indication of the immediate reversibility of air-flow obstruction.

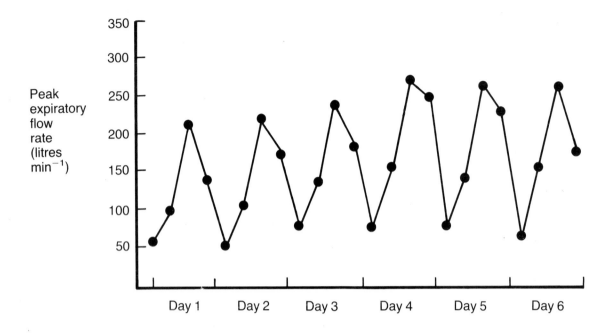

163 Peak flow monitoring showing 'morning dipping'. Frequent measurement of PEFR is useful in all asthmatic patients, but especially in those who show a diurnal variation in symptoms. The commonest problem is 'morning dipping', in which the patient's symptoms are worst in the early morning or on waking. This patient had only mild symptoms, but peak flow measurements showed severe, if variable, airflow obstruction, despite maintenance therapy with inhaled steroids and ß$_2$ agonists.

164

Respiratory function chart

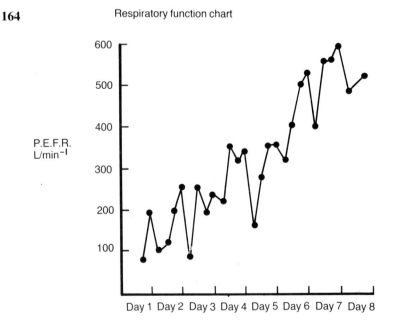

164 Peak flow monitoring showing successful therapy for acute asthma. This patient was admitted to hospital with severe pollen-induced asthma, and was treated initially with parenteral corticosteroids and ß$_2$ agonists, changing to a tapering dose of oral steroids and nebulised ß$_2$ agonists after the first 24 hours, and to inhaled steroids and ß$_2$ agonists before her discharge from hospital. Note the persistence of 'morning dipping'.

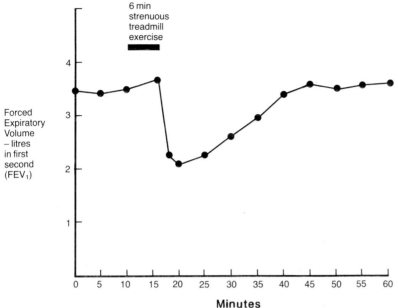

165 FEV$_1$ measurements in exercise-induced asthma. Six minutes of strenuous exercise on a treadmill results initially in a slight increase in FEV$_1$, but this is immediately followed by a substantial fall, accompanied by significant asthmatic symptoms. The mechanism of exercise-induced asthma is not completely clear; interestingly, it is often helped by 'anti-allergic' drugs such as sodium cromoglycate.

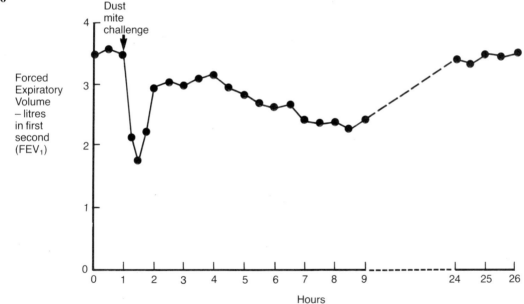

166 Bronchial challenge test in asthma, showing a biphasic response. Bronchial challenge tests are not without hazard, and require careful supervision, but they may occasionally be clinically useful, and they often show that a patient's asthma involves more than a simple type I reaction. Here, for example, there is an initial fall in FEV$_1$ which is consistent with a type I response. This is followed by recovery, but there is a later fall in FEV$_1$, accompanied by symptoms, which is not yet fully explained in immunological terms, but may be related to immune complex formation.

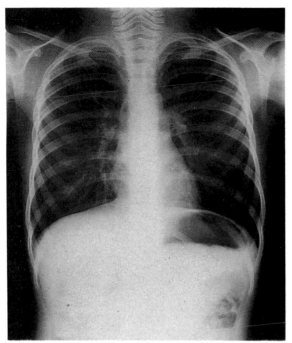

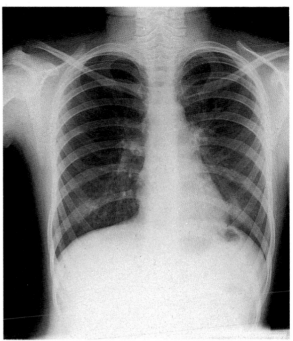

167 The chest xray is a poor guide to the severity of asthma. Although this 4-year-old girl had acute severe asthma requiring urgent treatment, her chest xray showed nothing more than mild hyperinflation.

168 Chronic asthma between attacks. The same patient as before—now aged 10. Again there are signs of mild hyperinflation of the chest, with perhaps slight prominence of the central blood vessels of the lungs, but otherwise the film is normal.

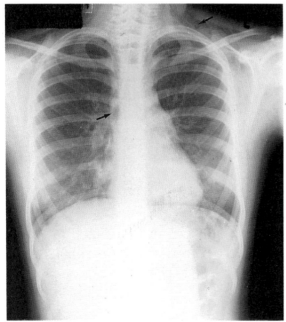

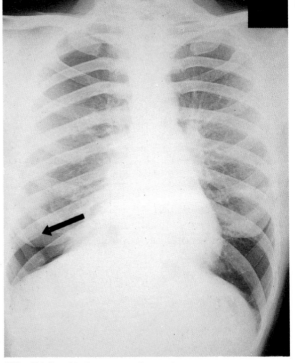

169 Pneumomediastinum, 'surgical' emphysema of the neck and a small pneumothorax in acute severe asthma. One year after the film in **168** was taken, the same girl was admitted with an attack of acute severe asthma which required urgent systemic steroid and bronchodilator treatment. Xray showed her to have a small right apical pneumothorax (difficult to see on this film). Air had also spread to her mediastinum (arrow) and the the soft tissue of her neck (arrow).

Pneumothorax is a frequent complication of acute asthma, but pneumomediastinum and 'surgical' emphysema are much less common. She made an uneventful recovery on treatment of her asthma, and no other treatment was required.

170 Right-sided pneumothorax in acute asthma in an adult. The edge of the collapsed lung is marked with an arrow. It is essential to consider the possibility of pneumothorax in those with severe acute asthma. This patient required urgent intercostal intubation in addition to systemic steroid and bronchodilator treatment.

ALLERGIC BRONCHOPULMONARY ASPERGILLOSIS

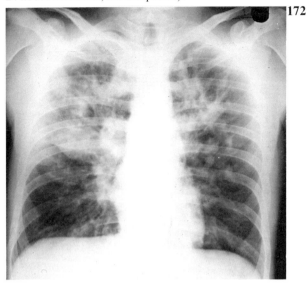

171

Species of the fungus *Aspergillus* are hardy and widespread in the environment—in soil, decaying vegetation, swimming pools and flour—and in house dust, bedding and damp walls and floors. The commonest species to infect man is *A. fumigatus*, and the individual's response is a clear example of the role of the immune status of the host in infection:

1 Aspergilloma, in which fungal infestation leads to a ball of fungus in the lung (a mycetoma) is commonest in non-atopic individuals with pre-existing lung cavities.

2 Locally invasive and systemic aspergillosis occur in patients with disease-induced or drug-induced immunosuppression.

3 Asthma may occur in atopic individuals where *Aspergillus* spores act in the same way as other inhaled allergens.

4 Extrinsic allergic bronchioalveolitis may rarely occur in both atopic and non-atopic individuals—the spores are small and can easily reach the periphery of the lung.

5 Allergic bronchopulmonary aspergillosis may occur in atopic patients. This disease follows a 'flu-like' illness which is accompanied by fleeting pulmonary consolidation, blood and/or sputum eosinophilia, copious mucus production and asthma—usually superimposed upon pre-existing extrinsic asthma. The patient shows an immediate positive skin-prick test to an extract of *A. fumigatus*. Late skin reactions may also occur, and specific precipitating antibodies to *A. fumigatus* are usually present in the serum. Recurrent attacks of eosinophilic pneumonia occur, and these usually lead to bronchiectasis.

171 Positive skin-prick test to aspergillus (E) in a patient with allergic bronchopulmonary aspergillosis. Note that the patient also has a positive response to grass pollen extract (C). The patient had pollen-induced asthma for many years before developing allergic bronchopulmonary aspergillosis (A: control; B: house dust mite; D: tree pollen).

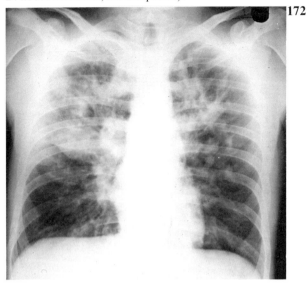

172

172 Allergic bronchopulmonary aspergillosis. Widespread non-segmental predominantly upper-zone shadows caused by eosinophilic pneumonia in a long-standing case of allergic aspergillosis. Malaise and fever are the usual symptoms, and blood eosinophilia accompanies the pulmonary consolidation.

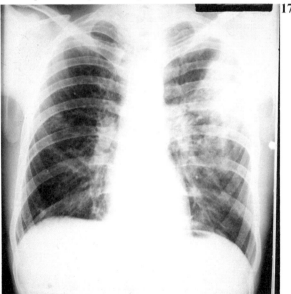

173

173 Allergic bronchopulmonary aspergillosis. Spontaneous clearing of most of the shadowing seen in **172** occurred within one month. The fleeting nature of the shadowing is often emphasised, but fixed abnormal shadows may be found. Bronchial plugs harbouring mycelial elements of the fungus block a segment of the left upper lobe.

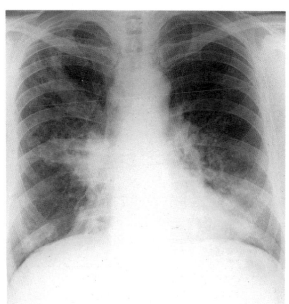

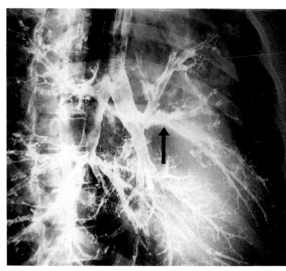

175 Bronchogram from a patient with bronchopulmonary aspergillosis showing characteristic proximal bronchiectasis. The arrow shows bronchial wall damage resulting from mucous plugging.

174 Bronchiectasis in allergic bronchopulmonary aspergillosis. Recurrent attacks of eosinophilic pneumonia with mucous plugging commonly result in bronchiectasis, as seen here in both upper lobes.

EOSINOPHILIC PNEUMONIA

Allergic bronchopulmonary aspergillosis is just one example of a number of disorders in which there is pulmonary disease in association with tissue and/or blood eosinophilia.

The radiological features are usually similar to those in acute allergic bronchopulmonary aspergillosis, and the symptoms are of variable severity (often mild).

A number of immunological and other mechanisms are probably involved in these reactions.

Where eosinophilic pneumonia is associated with parasite infestation (e.g. with ascariasis and in 'tropical eosinophilia' with microfilaria) type I reactions are often suggested by a massive rise in total IgE, but in other cases (e.g. Löeffler's syndrome) the mechanism is obscure.

Many drugs have been reported to cause pulmonary eosinophilia including nitrofurantoin, penicillins, sulphonamides, aspirin and antituberculous drugs.

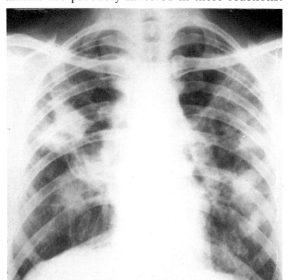

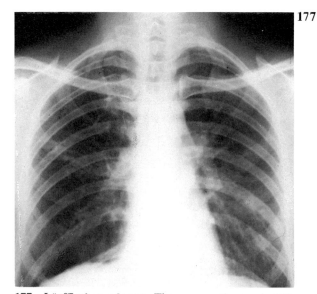

176 Löeffler's syndrome. The non-segmental transitory shadows tend to be distributed peripherally, giving an appearance sometimes called 'reverse pulmonary oedema'. In this patient, the total white cell count was 10,500 per mm^3 with 1600 (15 per cent) eosinophils.

177 Löeffler's syndrome. The same patient as in **176**, one month later. Spontaneous clearing of lung shadowing within a month is usual, but in this case clearing was accelerated by oral prednisolone.

EXTRINSIC ALLERGIC BRONCHIOALVEOLITIS (hypersensitivity pneumonitis)

Allergic bronchioalveolitis develops as a result of a hypersensitivity reaction in the lungs, and a wide range of organic dusts may provoke the condition. Many of these are encountered at work, and a large number of occupational lung diseases fall within this classification; while other causes relate to hobbies, especially the keeping of birds.

Repeated exposure of a susceptible individual to the offending antigen leads to the production of circulating precipitating antibodies and immune complexes (a type III reaction), and ultimately also to macrophage activation and epithelioid cell granuloma formation (type IV).

The factors which predispose to allergic bronchioalveolitis are poorly understood. There is some evidence of genetic susceptibility, but no link with atopy, or with elevated IgE or eosinophil levels.

Symptoms may develop within six hours of heavy exposure to the antigen, and the commonest presentation is with breathlessness, dry cough and influenza-like symptoms (malaise, fever and joint pains). Repeated exposure may lead to chronic respiratory impairment due to fibrosis of the lungs—in fact, to abnormalities identical with those seen in cryptogenic fibrosing alveolitis.

Table 32. Some of the commonest causes of extrinsic allergic bronchiolar-alveolitis in the UK

Disease	Provoking activity	Antigens
Farmer's lung	Forking mouldy vegetable matter, especially mouldy hay	Thermophilic actinomycetes *Micropolyspora faeni*
Bird fancier's lung	Handling pigeons or cleaning pigeon lofts and budgerigar cages	Proteins from feathers and excreta
Maltworker's lung	Turning germinating barley	*Aspergillus clavatus*
Humidifier fever	Working in offices or factories with contaminated air-conditioning or humidifying systems	Possibly bacterial or protozoal (esp *Naegleria gruberi*)

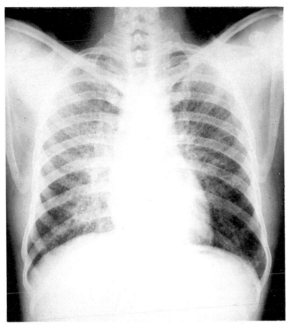

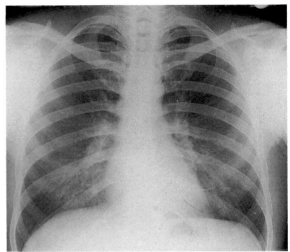

179 Pigeon fancier's lung. This man presented with acute symptoms after cleaning out his pigeon loft. The xray shows diffuse, hazy opacification in both lung fields which partially obscures the normal vascular markings.

178 Acute farmer's lung. Caused principally by *Micropolyspora faeni* in mouldy hay, though other fungi are also important in some cases. Fine nodular shadows are visible in the central two-thirds of the chest xray. In mild attacks there may be no lung function abnormality, but in severe attacks there is a restrictive defect.

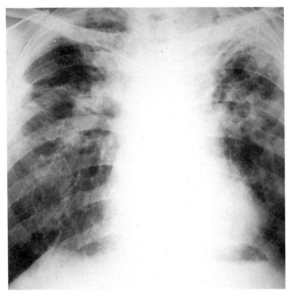

180 Budgerigar fancier's lung. Budgerigar fanciers may develop similar xray changes to pigeon fanciers (**179**), but because they often keep their birds indoors, their exposure to antigen is more constant and they usually present with insidious chronic lung diseases. This xray shows upper lobe fibrosis and bullae, which have led to a permanent severe ventilatory restriction and diffusion defect.

OTHER LUNG DISEASES

As the table on page 73 shows, immunological abnormalities may be present in a range of diseases of the lungs; and systemic autoimmune disorders such as SLE and rheumatoid arthritis may also have pulmonary manifestations. In some lung diseases, detectable immunological abnormalities may be an 'epiphenomenon', while in others they may be secondary to other as yet undetected causes, such as infection.

Most of these disorders involve type III and/or type IV reactions, and may improve on treatment with corticosteroids or immunosuppressive drugs. Only the rare Goodpasture's syndrome involves a type II (cytotoxic) reaction, while none of these disorders clearly involve type I (immediate hypersensitivity) reactions.

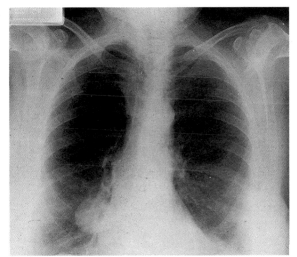

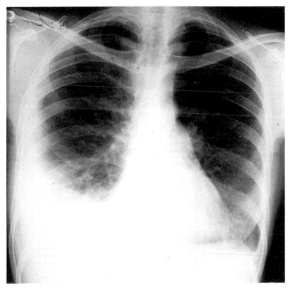

181 Rheumatoid nodule in the right lower lobe of a 55-year-old woman with rheumatoid arthritis. The precise site was confirmed by a lateral xray. This sharply defined spherical lesion grew slowly over a period of five years. Rheumatoid nodules are more common in male patients, and solitary nodules often require biopsy to exclude malignancy. Histologically, rheumatoid nodules have a central area of fibrinoid necrosis, surrounded by chronic inflammatory cells. Note the rheumatoid changes in the left shoulder joint.

182 Rheumatoid pleural effusion in male patient. Rheumatoid effusions contain predominantly lymphocytes, and may precede joint symptoms.

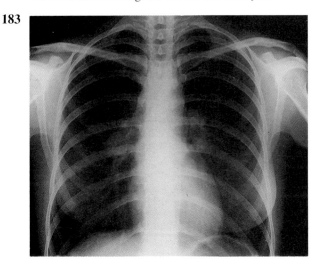

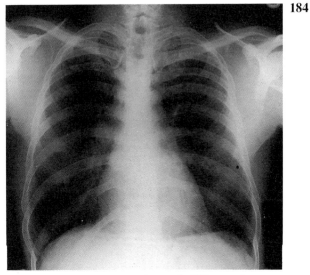

183 Sarcoidosis. This chest xray shows bilateral hilar and paratracheal lymphadenopathy in a 25-year-old woman who presented with erythema nodosum (see Figure **84**). The aetiology of sarcoidosis is unknown. Its immunological features include a depression of delayed-type hypersensitivity (T-cell anergy) and an elevation of serum immunoglobulins (B-cell hyperactivity).

184 Hilar lymphadenopathy and diffuse pulmonary infiltration in sarcoidosis. The diffuse infiltration is obvious bilaterally in the upper and mid-zones, and histological confirmation was obtained by biopsy through a fibreoptic bronchoscope.

8 GASTROINTESTINAL TRACT AND FOOD ALLERGIES

The gut is an active immunological organ, and an immune response to food—commonly involving local IgA-based mechanisms—is part of the body's normal reaction to the 'foreign' material it contains.

In recent years, 'food allergy' has become a fashionable diagnosis. A wide variety of gastrointestinal and remote symptoms has been attributed to an abnormal allergic response to foods. The evidence for this link is tenuous or absent in most cases, however, and a true allergic response to food is relatively uncommon.

Ingested allergens undoubtedly play a part in the symptoms of some patients with other signs of atopy, such as atopic eczema (particularly in children), urticaria, rhinitis or asthma, but their role in patients with psychiatric disorders or multiple vague symptomatology is unproven.

A number of symptoms and syndromes can be clearly related to food and food additives; it is clear that both gastrointestinal and remote disorders may result from food intolerance in a number of ways, most of which do not directly involve immunological reactions. The true mechanisms are poorly understood in many cases, but they may involve idiosyncratic reactions or direct reactions to pharmacologically active substances in ingested food. Sometimes histamine and other vasoactive substances are released, and the reaction closely resembles a type I allergic response. Some reactions which have in the past been regarded as classical allergic responses (e.g. urticaria following the ingestion of strawberries) are probably the result of direct vasoactive amine release rather than a true allergic response. The practical significance of this distinction is not great at present, as the principles of management of these conditions are usually similar regardless of the underlying mechanism.

Even where immunological abnormalities or allergic reactions have been demonstrated clearly—as, for example, in gluten-sensitive enteropathy—it is often not clear whether these are involved in the primary disease process, or whether they are simply a secondary consequence of other initiating factors.

Table 33. Symptoms and syndromes which may be related to food

Gastrointestinal symptoms	Swelling of lips or mouth
	Oral ulceration
	Vomiting
	Diarrhoea
	Abdominal pain
	Bloating
	Constipation
	Pruritus ani
Secondary syndromes	Steatorrhoea and 'coeliac-like' syndromes
	Protein-losing enteropathy
	Blood loss and anaemia (rare)
	Eosinophilic gastroenteritis
Remote effects	Anaphylaxis
	Rhinitis
	Nasal polyps
	Asthma
	Eczema
	Urticaria and angioedema
	Dermatitis herpetiformis
	Transitory joint pains
	Migraine
	Hyperactivity in children (food association very rare)
	Henoch-Schönlein purpura (rare)
	Nephrotic syndrome (rare)

CLINICAL FEATURES OF FOOD INTOLERANCE

Where foods regularly provoke gastrointestinal symptoms, the patient will often suspect an association, and this may also be the case where a rarely eaten food produces a dramatic response. Where the food is a part of the everyday diet, the association may be less obvious, but the possibility of food intolerance should be considered in all patients with:

- urticaria and angioedema
- atopic eczema
- migraine
- asthma
- rhinitis

In rhinitis with nasal polyps, intolerance to aspirin may also be present.

The manifestations of food intolerance may be immediate or delayed. Symptoms such as swelling of lips and tongue, urticaria, vomiting, rhinorrhoea and asthma often develop within minutes as a result of an IgE-mediated reaction or a direct pharmacological effect. Late reactions may develop some hours or even days after ingestion of food, possibly as a result of a delayed immune response involving circulating immune complexes. Such late reactions pose a particularly difficult diagnostic problem.

Table 34.   Causes of food intolerance

Pharmacological
Caffeine
Tyramine—e.g. in cheese
Histamine—e.g. in fish and canned foods
Histamine liberators—e.g. egg white, strawberries
Nitrates—e.g. in preserved meat

Toxic
Irritants of the intestinal mucosa—e.g. peppers and spices
Poisons—e.g. from tropical sea fish; acetanilide
  in rape-seed oil; aflatoxin in mouldy peanuts

Idiosyncracy
Deficiency of enzymes e.g. lactase (cow's milk intolerance) and possbily phenolsulphotransferase (some cases of dietary migraine)

Indirect associations
Fat intolerance due to gall bladder disease, cystic fibrosis or steatorrhoea
Intolerance to fried or spiced foods in peptic ulceration
Irritable bowel syndrome (possible effects of fermentation of unabsorbed food residues)

Food allergic disease
IgE-mediated—usually associated with other allergies
Other immunological abnormalities—e.g. coeliac disease, cow's milk and soya protein intolerance in infants

---

Table 35.   Investigations in suspected food intolerance

- There are no reliable laboratory tests for food allergy or idiosyncracy.

- Skin-prick testing with a few food extracts such as egg, fish, nuts and yeast gives results which correlate well with clinical symptoms, but positive results tend to persist even when clinical sensitivity has been lost.

- Serum IgE may be raised in an allergic response, but this does not demonstrate that the responsible antigen entered via the gut.

- Radioallergosorbent tests (RASTs) for specific IgE antibodies may sometimes demonstrate raised circulating antibody levels to specific foods, but for most of the food extracts used the correlation with symptoms is poor.

- 'Fringe' techniques, such as sublingual or cytotoxic food tests, hair analysis, etc, are widely advertised but valueless.

- A diagnostic exclusion diet, followed by appropriate food challenge, is the mainstay of investigation.

DIAGNOSTIC AND THERAPEUTIC EXCLUSION DIETS

A 'full exclusion diet' is very restricted. The precise content varies from one centre to another, but the common aim is to exclude all foods which could provoke symptoms. Many patients find it difficult to adhere to a full exclusion diet, and for some conditions it is possible to use a less restricted diet in the first instance, following this with a period on a full exclusion diet if necessary.

The patient should keep a detailed food diary throughout the exclusion period. If the symptoms do not remit during 2-3 weeks on this diet, food or food additives are an unlikely cause of symptoms. Futher investigation and/or symptomatic treatments are then indicated.

If the symptoms remit on the diet, the patient should reintroduce all the excluded foods one at a time, (at intervals of 2-7 days) over the next few months, while continuing on a gradually expanding exclusion diet throughout this period (composed of the original diet together with additional foods as they are shown not to cause symptoms). Foods should be introduced in order of importance in a normal diet—e.g. tap water first, followed by potatoes, cow's milk, yeast etc—but if the patient suspects individual excluded foods of causing symptoms, these should be reintroduced early in the second phase, as a response to their reintroduction may make further investigation unnecessary.

The role of individual foods can be confirmed by the 'blind' administration of freeze-dried food in unmarked capsules, so that the patient is unaware of the nature of the food under test. This technique has a limitation of small volume, which should not affect true allergic responses, but may prevent adverse responses of other kinds. It also prevents the food from coming into contact with the lips, mouth and oesophagus, and may not reproduce symptoms related to these organs. In practice, the technique is usually reserved for formal studies, and despite its recent surge in popularity in the USA, it has a limited role in routine investigation.

Table 36. The management of food intolerance

- Isolated reactions to foods which can be avoided (strawberries, shellfish, etc) are best managed by simple avoidance.

- Multiple intolerance—especially when it involves intolerance to cow's milk, eggs, yeast, etc—can be managed by a more rigorous therapeutic exclusion diet, but this must be carefully planned and monitored to ensure nutritional adequacy, and compliance with the diet is often a problem.

- Desensitisation therapy using injections, or by oral or nasal administrarion, has been advocated by some, but the evidence of success for well-publicised techniques such as sublingual drop treatment is almost totally unscientific.

- There is no specific drug treatment for food allergy or idiosyncracy, though oral sodium cromoglycate may have occasional value as an adjunct to diet in multiple food allergy. The appropriate dose of the drug is not known, and probably varies widely from one patient to another.

- Adverse responses to food may change with time, and problem foods should be reintroduced on a trial basis at intervals.

- Coeliac disease is a special case, requiring prolonged treatment with a gluten-free diet.

- Symptomatic treatment of asthma, rhinitis, eczema, migraine, etc, is often necessary and effective; and it may be preferable to a prolonged exclusion diet and/or a useful additional part of therapy.

Table 37. Diagnostic exclusion diets appropriate for possibly food-related symptoms*

Condition	Diagnostic diet
Urticaria or angioedema	Tartrazine and salicylate free
Eczema	Cow's milk and egg free
Coeliac disease	Gluten free
Cow's milk sensitive enteropathy	Cow's milk free
Asthma and rhinitis	Full exclusion
Migraine	Full exclusion
Irritable bowel syndrome	Full exclusion

---

*A full exclusion diet should be tried if a more specific diet is unsuccessful.

FOOD INTOLERANCE AND THE SKIN

Cases of eczema, urticaria and angioedema provoked by food intolerance cannot be distinguished on clinical examination from those resulting from other causes. Food or food additives should always be considered, though most cases of eczema and many cases of urticaria and angioedema have other causes or no identifiable cause.

It is impractical to use diagnostic exclusion diets in all cases, and they should usually be reserved for those patients who (or whose parents) strongly suspect a food-related cause, for those with continuous or recurrent severe symptoms, and for those who have experienced episodic asthma, laryngeal oedema or anaphylaxis in association with angioedema.

Food intolerance may contribute to eczema of the types illustrated in **25-30**, and may provoke urticaria and angioedema as shown in **52, 57** and **59**.

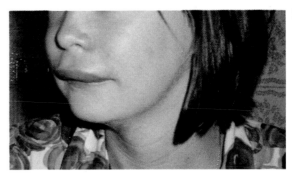

186   Angioedema resulting from tartrazine sensitivity. This girl had recurrent, severe angioedema and urticaria, with episodes of life-threatening laryngeal oedema. An exclusion diet showed tartrazine (E102) to be the cause of her symptoms. This food colouring is widely used in many processed foods and drinks, so a rigorous maintenance exclusion diet is required to prevent symptoms. The mechanism of tartrazine sensitivity is unclear, and it may not have an allergic basis. Cross sensitivity with other azo dyes and with aspirin is common.

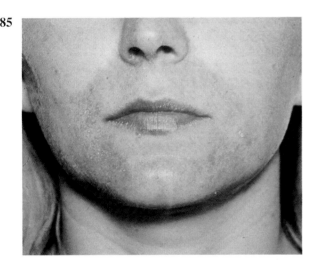

185   Eczema resulting from orange drink. The patient suspected the cause, and the perioral distribution of the lesions suggested a contact or ingested cause. An exclusion diet showed the cause to be the food-colouring azo dyes tartrazine (E102) and sunset yellow (E110), and not orange juice itself (but note that citrus fruits are among the commoner causes of food-related symptoms).

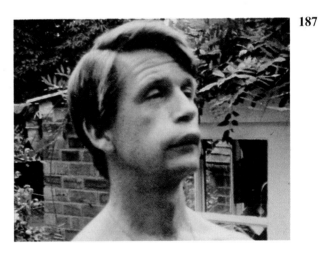

187   Angioedema resulting from salicylate sensitivity. This man avoided taking aspirin because he knew that it provoked severe angioedema and asthma, but he continued to suffer from recurrent attacks—as shown here. These resulted from his sensitivity to salicylates in natural and processed foods. They may occur naturally in many fruits, wine, vinegar and liquorice, and as an additive in foods such as jam, jelly, ice cream, chewing gum and soft drinks. An appropriate exclusion diet prevented all but the occasional attack, and the remaining attacks of angioedema—due to unavoidable exposure—have responded to antihistamine therapy.

188

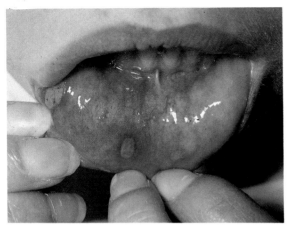

189

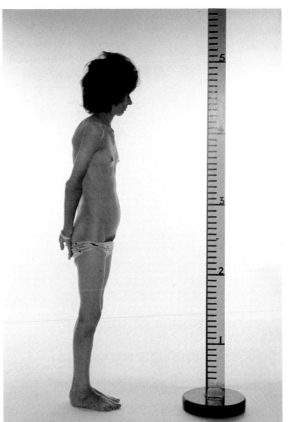

188 Aphthous ulceration. This is common but the cause is unknown, though many cases probably result from trauma with superimposed infection. Food intolerance may be an occasional contributory factor, but there is no evidence of food intolerance in most cases. Similar, but more severe, ulceration occurs in Behçet's syndrome and other systemic mucocutaneous disorders, where there are undoubted immunological abnormalities—but there is no evidence for an allergic mechanism. Aphthous ulceration cannot be regarded as an allergic condition.

190

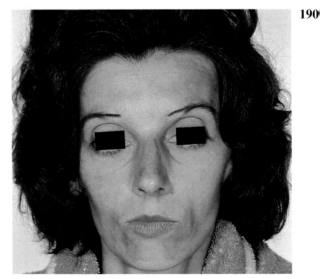

189 and 190 Coeliac disease. Gluten intolerance may remain undiagnosed for many years. This woman was diagnosed at the age of 32, but her height (5'0"—lower than all other members of her family) suggests that her malabsorption dates from childhood. At presentation she weighed 40 kg (88 pounds), she had marked steatorrhoea and she was pale and anaemic. Small bowel biopsy showed villous atrophy.

A gluten-free diet relieved her steatorrhoea and reversed the changes in her jejunal mucosa. She rapidly gained weight, but should probably remain on a gluten-free diet for life.

Gluten-sensitive enteropathy

In coeliac disease the small bowel is sensitive to gluten, and a jejunal biopsy demonstrates villous atrophy of the small bowel mucosa. Histology shows infiltration of the submucosa by lymphocytes, eosinophils and plasma cells. Similar findings occur in most patients with dermatitis herpetiformis.

There is clear evidence of immunological abnormalities in coeliac disease, including circulating antigliadin antibodies in most patients, antireticulin antibodies in 50 per cent, and a range of other abnormalities. There is also an increase in malignancy.

It seems likely that these immunological abnormalities are involved in the primary cause of the disease, but the mechanism is not clear, and it is still possible that gluten induces initial damage by non-immunological means, and that the immunological abnormalities are a secondary phenomenon.

A gluten-free diet relieves symptoms and reverses the small bowel changes in both coeliac disease and dermatitis herpetiformis—though the skin eruption in dermatitis herpetiformis often responds slowly and dapsone treatment may be required as well.

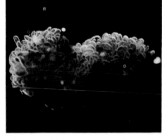 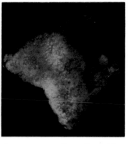

192 and 193 Jejunal biopsies from normal and coeliac patients. Seen here under the dissecting microscope immediately after removal from the Crosby capsule.

The normal mucosa (**192**) shows a normal pattern and number of jejunal villi, whereas the abnormal mucosa (**193**) shows complete flattening—the characteristic appearance of gluten-sensitive enteropathy.

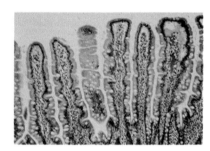

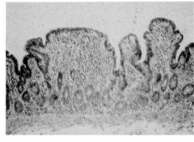

194 and 195 Microscopic sections of jejunal biopsies from normal and coeliac patients. The sections correspond to the macroscopic appearances seen in **192** and **193** respectively. Figure **194** shows the normal microscopic appearance of the jejunal mucosa, as seen in a healthy individual.

By contrast, **195** shows the jejunum of a previously undiagnosed patient with gluten-sensitive enteropathy on a normal diet. The normal intestinal villi are absent, the mucosa is flattened, and there is hyperplasia of the intestinal crypts. There is lymphocytic infiltration, and the surface mucosa is cuboidal rather than columnar (as in **194**)—this mucosal change reflecting the impaired function of the intestinal mucosa in gluten-sensitive enteropathy.

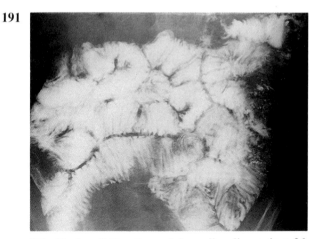

191 Barium follow-through in coeliac disease in a 26-year-old man. The film shows dilatation of the small bowel with 'simplification' of the mucosal pattern—the transverse folds are straight in appearance, rather than 'feathery' as they would be in normal film. Flocculation of barium used to be described as a classic sign of coeliac disease, but the additives in modern barium prevent this sign from appearing. Nevertheless, the diagnosis is suggested clearly by the film.

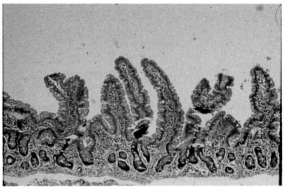

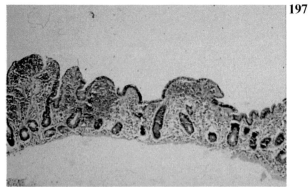

196 **The jejunal mucosa in treated coeliac disease.** The adoption of a gluten-free diet in coeliac disease usually restores the jejunal mucosa to normal within three months, but the bowel generally remains gluten sensitive for life (see **197** and **199**). This continuing sensitivity is a powerful reason for a lifelong gluten-free diet in most patients, although it is not yet clear whether gluten avoidance reduces the increased risk of gastrointestinal malignancy which accompanies the disease.

197 **Gluten challenge in a patient with treated coeliac disease rapidly damages the intestinal mucosa.** This section was taken from the same patient as **196**. Immediately after that biopsy was obtained the patient was given an oral gluten challenge. This biopsy was taken just six hours after the gluten challenge, but shows essentially the same changes as in the long-term coeliac (see **195**).

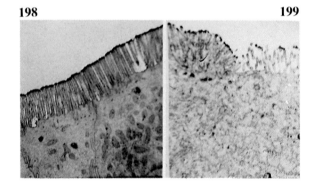

198 and 199 **Electron microscopy of the mucosal cells before and six hours after gluten challenge in a patient with coeliac disease shows the acute damage inflicted by gluten in this condition.** The mucosal cell in **198** has a normal brush border and its cytoplasm contains normal organelles. By contrast, in the post-challenge cell (**199**) the brush border is destroyed and the cytoplasm shows few recognisable features.

Inflammatory bowel disease

Milk-induced colitis in infants seems to have an allergic basis, but, despite many suggestions over the past 50 years, it seems unlikely that allergic reactions are in any way causative in adult inflammatory bowel disease. Circulating antibodies to food and circulating immune complexes may often be found, but these may well be a secondary consequence of intestinal mucosal damage rather than a primary factor.

Milk intolerance is a problem in some patients with ulcerative colitis and Crohn's disease, but it can usually be explained by hypolactasia rather than allergy.

It has been suggested that a high intake of refined sugar and a low intake of dietary fibre may be a factor in the genesis of Crohn's disease, but the evidence for this suggestion is not firm; there is no evidence for an allergic mechanism, though there is evidence that intolerance to foods may influence symptoms in some patients. The use of elemental diets may decrease gastrointestinal protein loss in Crohn's disease, but it seems unlikely that withdrawal of dietary allergens plays any part in the resulting improvement.

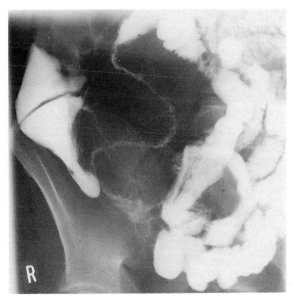

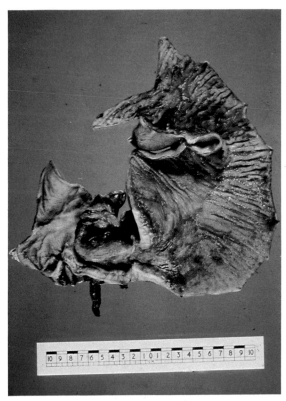

200 and 201 Ileal Crohn's disease. The barium follow through (**200**) shows a long stricture of the terminal ileum, surrounded by a soft tissue mass which can be seen to indent the caecum. Figure **201** shows the terminal ileum of another patient resected at surgery. Note the presence of a similar stricture in the terminal ileum.

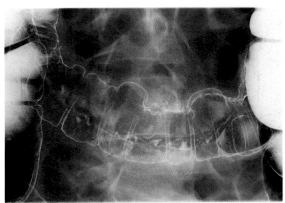

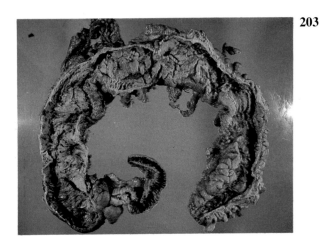

202 and 203 Colonic Crohn's disease. The double contrast barium enema (**202**) shows a number of deep ulcers in the transverse colon, characteristic of Crohn's disease. The remaining mucosa is normal. These 'skip lesions' in which only part of the circumference and length of the bowel is affected, help differentiate colonic Crohn's disease from ulcerative colitis.

The resected colon (**203**—from another patient) again shows skip lesions, with normal areas of colon between them.

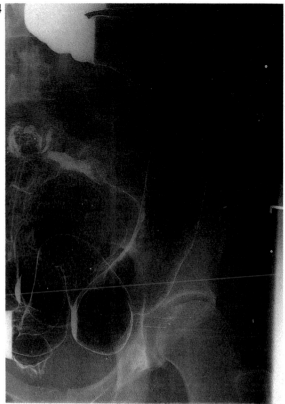

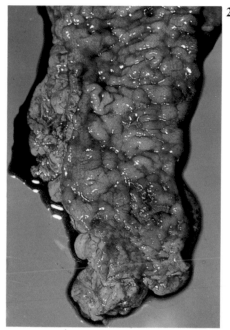

throughout the entire colon. This represents a destruction of the mucosa, revealing the bare muscularis mucosae, which is studded with islands of regenerating mucosa.

The resection specimen (**205**) shows the macroscopic appearance of a severely affected colon. The mucosa is friable and haemorrhagic, and the regenerating islands of mucosa have the appearance of 'pseudopolyps'.

204 and 205   Ulcerative colitis. The double contrast barium enema (**204**) shows a continuous fine granularity of the descending colon, which, in fact, extended

ALLERGY AND THE LIVER

Though immunological abnormalities are present in a number of liver diseases, few, if any, are true 'allergic' disorders. Most of the immunological abnormalities are probably a consequence of other initiating processes, especially infection, and some are of doubtful authenticity—e.g. there is no firm evidence that any drug induces immunologically mediated liver damage.

One possible 'allergic' disorder is primary biliary cirrhosis. The aetiology of the disease is unknown, but the bile duct damage seems to be immunologically mediated. Seventy per cent of patients have a polyclonal increase in serum IgM level and IgG and IgA levels may also be increased. Antimitochondrial antibodies are present in the serum of over 95 per cent of patients. Some patients have associated Sjögren's syndrome or other connective tissue disorders (see Chapter 9).

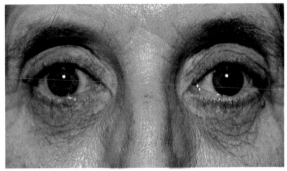

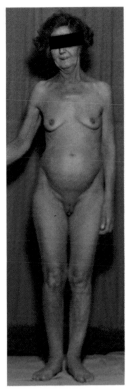

206 and 207 Primary biliary cirrhosis. This 55-year-old woman presented originally with severe pruritus, and jaundice developed slowly over the next three years. When these photographs were taken she had deep jaundice, spider naevi, xanthelasmata around both eyes, enlargement of the liver and spleen and ascites. Sadly, the deepening jaundice and ascites are poor prognostic signs, and are usually followed by encephalopathy and death within weeks or months.

FOOD INTOLERANCE AND THE KIDNEY

As with the liver, many diseases of the kidney involve immunological processes of Type III, and some involve Type II and Type IV reactions, but in few, if any, are Type I allergic processes a primary event. One possible example is the nephrotic syndrome, in which immediate allergic reactions may sometimes play a part. The number of documented cases is small, but it seems possible that nephrotic syndrome (usually 'minimal change' on biopsy) may rarely result from allergy to cow's milk, eggs and indeed also to inhaled allergens such as pollen and moulds. The evidence for this view results from studies involving challenge with, and withdrawal of, cow's milk, and from densensitisation studies in some of the pollen–sensitive patients. It is not yet clear whether Type I reactions account for a larger number of cases of minimal change nephrotic syndrome—or indeed for other renal diseases, but the possibility has important therapeutic implications.

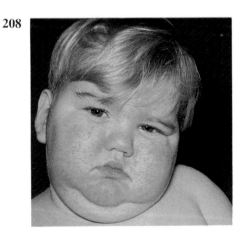

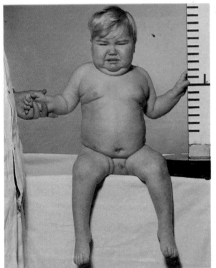

208 and 209 Nephrotic syndrome in a 2½-year-old boy. His severe facial and body oedema resulted from his gross proteinuria and hypoproteinaemia. Renal biopsy showed minimal change glomerulonephritis and he was treated with steroids to good effect, ultimately going into complete remission. Idiopathic nephrotic syndrome is usually steroid responsive, and this response does not prove a type I aetiology.

9   AUTOIMMUNE DISEASES

The marker common to all autoimmune diseases is the presence of humoral autoantibodies. These probably reflect more basic defects of the immune system such as the loss of T lymphocyte suppressor activity. Immune complex damage is variable and is sometimes a secondary phenomenon. There is a failure to suppress the response to self antigens. Foreign antigens from microbes or drugs may share epitopes with self antigens. The unshared part of the foreign antigens may then bypass T cell tolerance and in that way gain T lymphocyte recognition, so stimulating a clone of B lymphocytes which react with both foreign and 'self' components. HLA DR3 seems to be associated with several conditions (see Table 38). Possibly a gene linked to that for DR3 increases immune responsiveness.

Autoimmunity may affect single or multiple organs. Overlap between conditions occur and the aetiology is usually known. The presence of autoantibodies may be demonstrated by a number of techniques (see Tables 7 and 8).

LUPUS ERYTHEMATOSUS SYNDROME (LE)
Discoid LE

Discoid lupus should not be confused with the systemic variety in which general health is affected and major laboratory abnormalities are found. The skin is always affected in discoid lupus, but it is not always affected in the systemic form. Progression from discoid to systemic lupus erythematosus is rare.

Treatment of discoid lupus must include strict sun avoidance and the use of sunscreens. Topical steroids and, in resistant cases, a short course of antimalarial therapy—e.g. hydroxychloroquine—may be used for a short time during the summer months only to avoid eye complications.

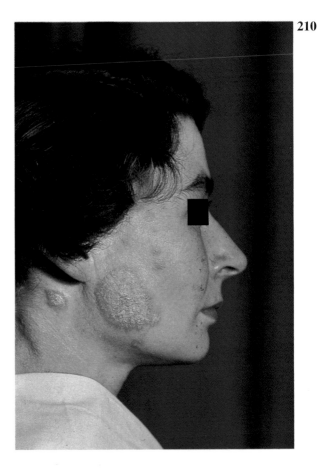

210

210   Discoid lupus erythematosus. Slowly enlarging recalcitrant pink scaly plaques seen on the face, ears and scalp.

Table 38.   Diseases in which HLA DR3 may be associated with autoimmune reactions

---

- Systemic lupus erythematosus
- Sjögren's syndrome
- Addison's disease
- Chronic hepatitis
- Myasthenia gravis
- Graves' disease

211 Discoid lupus erythematosus. Lesions are aggravated by sunlight and clear centrally with atrophy and scarring.

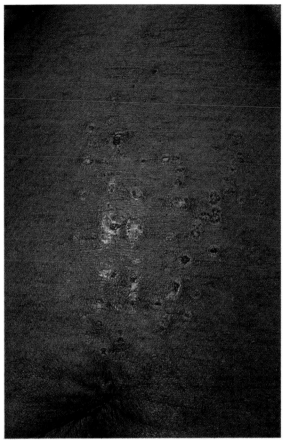

212 Follicular plugging in discoid lupus erythematosus. Characteristically the scales are follicular. Rarely the condition may be widespread or disseminated.

Systemic LE

Cutaneous signs of SLE include a butterfly rash on the face, frontal alopecia which is non-scarring, mucosal ulceration, nail fold telangiectasia and erythema, Raynaud's phenomenon and discrete palpable purpuric lesions signifying vasculitis. Patients often present with systemic symptoms such as malaise, fever and arthralgia. The aetiology is usually unknown, but the disease may be drug induced, especially in slow acetylators. Treatment involves systemic steroids or immunosuppressive drugs.

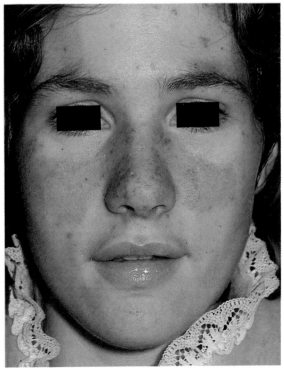

213 Systemic lupus erythematosus (SLE). The characteristic 'butterfly' rash in a 17-year-old female patient.

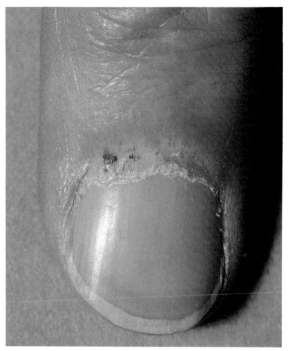

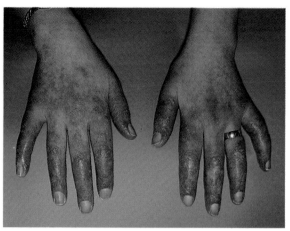

215 Raynaud's phenomenon is a common ac-companying symptom in SLE, involving hands and feet. Rarely gangrene can occur.

214 Nail fold erythema and telangiectasia with ragged cuticles. This is often seen in SLE, but also in other non-organ-specific autoimmune disorders such as dermatomyositis.

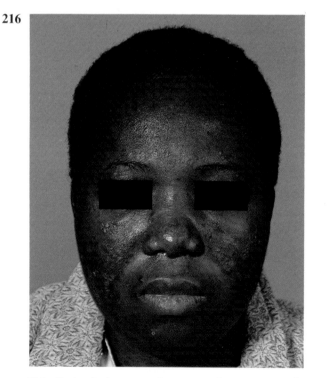

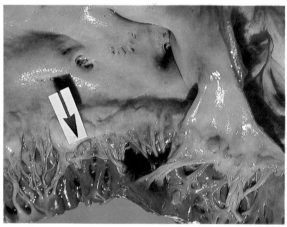

217 Cardiac involvement in SLE includes immune complex deposition and (arrowed) thickening of the heart valves (Libman-Sacks endocarditis). It can simu-late rheumatic heart disease.

216 Systemic lupus erythematosus is commonest in black women of child-bearing age such as this 33-year-old West Indian woman who presented with a rash over her cheeks.

Table 39. Lupus erythematosus syndrome

	Discoid lupus erythematosus	Systemic lupus erthematosus
Sex ratio (F:M)	2:1	8:1
Age (commonest)	wide range	30s
Photosensitivity	50%	20%
Skin	erythema, hyperkeratosis, follicular plugging, telangiectasia	macular erythema, butterfly rash, telangiectasia
Scarring	+	–
Immunofluorescence (lupus band test)	+ (abnormal skin)	+ (all skin)
Antinuclear factor	30%	100%
Antibody to double stranded DNA	usually negative	high titre in 80% +
Circulating LE cells	0	70 - 80%
Serum Complement	normal	normal or low
Rheumatoid factor	0	2C - 40%
Antibody to extractable nuclear antigen	0	20%

218 The lupus band test demonstrates the deposition of complement and immunoglobulin in the skin at the dermoepidermal junction, shown here as a continuous band of IgM (arrow) by direct immunofluorescence (the background fluorescence in the dermis is not significant in this context). Non-lesional, light-exposed skin should be used for this test. See also page 23.

Table 40. Preliminary criteria for the classification of systemic lupus erythematosus*

	American Rheumatism Association % incidence	UK % incidence
Facial erythema	64	62
Discoid lupus	17	30
Raynaud's phenomenon	20	19
Alopecia	43	62
Photosensitivity	37	16
Oral/nasopharyngeal ulceration	15	22
Arthritis without deformity	90	86
LE Cells	92	73
Chronic false positive serological tests for syphilis	12	8
Proteinuria 3.5 g per 24 h	20	24
Cellular casts in urine	48	16
Pleuritis and/or pericarditis	60/19	30/19
Psychosis and/or convulsions	19	19
Haematological abnormalities one or more of:		
haemolytic anaemia	16	14
leucopenia	40	46
thrombocytopenia	11	14

*A positive score of four or more of the criteria shown here confirms the diagnosis of systemic lupus erythematosus.

Table 41. Drugs which may induce a systemic lupus erythematosus-like syndrome

Frequently
Hydrallazine
Procainamide
Isoniazid
Phenothiazine
Oral contraceptives*

Rarely
L-dopa
d-Penicillamine
Phenylbutazone
Reserpine
Quinidine
Cotrimoxaole*
Penicillin*

*May also exacerbate existing SLE.

Features of drug-induced SLE: (1) renal and central nervous systems are rarely involved; (2) the syndrome resolves on withdrawal of the offending drug.

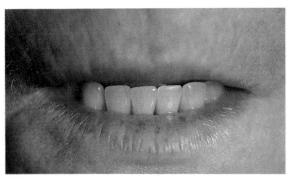

220 Progressive systemic sclerosis (scleroderma) with characteristic telangiectasia and radial furrowing around the mouth. Eventually the face becomes waxy and mask-like.

Progressive systemic sclerosis
In contrast to morphoea this is a serious multi-system disease. Patients are usually female. They present with Raynaud's phenomenon and/or dysphagia. The heart, lungs, kidney and gastro-intestinal tract may be involved. Occasionally a fulminating variety leads to rapid death. Positive investigations include high titres of antinuclear factor and abnormal oesophageal motility. Also lung, liver and renal function may be affected. Treatment is disappointing. Potassium aminobenzoate, penicillamine and systemic corticosteroids have been used in therapy with varying results. Physiotherapy and thermoregulation are often helpful in symptomatic relief, as is cimetidine for symptoms of oesophageal reflux.

SCLERODERMA

Morphoea
This is a localised form of scleroderma. Rarely the growth of underlying structures may be affected. Often spontaneous resolution occurs. No treatment is helpful.

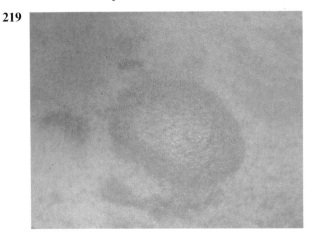

219 Morphoea of the abdomen. This presents as erythematous plaques with an advancing violaceous border. When inactive they become indurated, white and later brown.

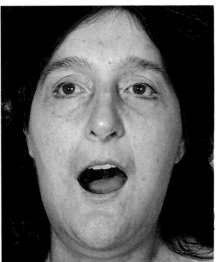

221 Characteristic facies of systemic sclerosis with limited opening of the mouth.

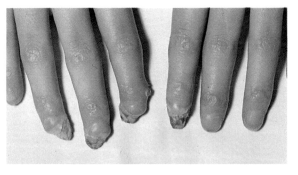

222 Calcinosis cutis and sclerodactyly occur in digits with severe Raynaud's phenomenon, causing ischaemia and gangrene.

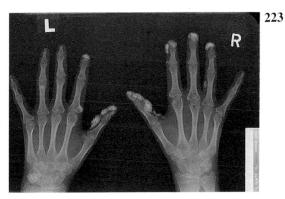

223 Extensive subcutaneous and soft tissue calcification shown on xray in scleroderma.

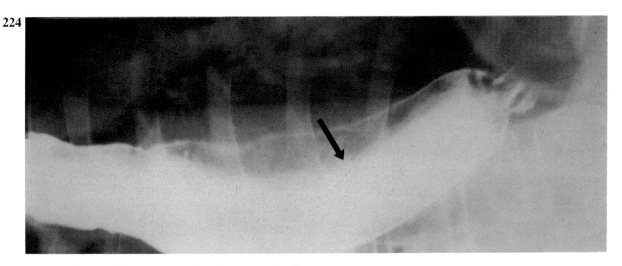

224 Barium swallow may reveal reflux oesophagitis and subsequent stricture due to oesophageal hypomobility from systemic sclerosis which often occurs early in the disease. Supine films may show a fluid level (arrowed), demonstrating oesophageal rigidity.

DERMATOMYOSITIS

This is a rare condition which may be associated with an underlying malignancy—usually an adenocarcinoma. Apart from cutaneous manifestations, proximal muscle weakness and pain occur due to a polymyositis. Electromyography and muscle biopsy may aid diagnosis. Serum creatine phosphokinase is usually elevated. Hyper-gammaglobulinaemia, rheumatoid factor, antinuclear factor and false positive tests for syphilis can occasionally be found (see Table 42).

If no obvious tumour is found, prostate, breasts and pelvic organs should be investigated—sadly, most underlying tumours are not easily treatable.

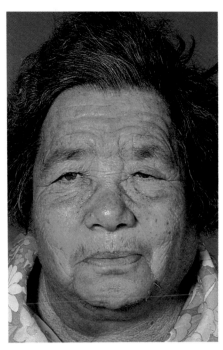

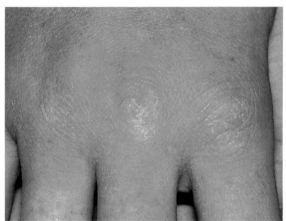

226 Violaceous plaques and papules may occur on the knuckles, knees and elbows in dermatomyositis. This picture shows erythematous streaking over the extensor tendons of the hands.

225 Dermatomyositis. This usually affects patients over 40 years of age. There is characteristic erythema and oedema of the face with slight purple discoloration of the eyelids.

POLYARTERITIS NODOSA

Patients with polyarteritis nodosa (PAN) are usually ill and febrile, with a cutaneous vasculitis. PAN is a multisystem disorder and other signs and symptoms result from the involvement of the renal, abdominal, coronary, respiratory and central nervous system vasculature. Investigations may reveal elevated ESR, gammaglobulin level, e.g. $\propto 2$ globulin, leucocytosis, eosinophilia and anaemia. Diagnosis can be confirmed by identifying vessel involvement by radiological techniques and by biopsy of arterioles where indicated. Treatment includes immunosuppresive drugs and systemic corticosteroids.

Recently a cutaneous form of PAN without systemic involvement has been described. It consists of palpable nodes and livedo reticularis usually over the legs, rarely associated with neuropathy and myalgia. Prognosis for this variant is very good.

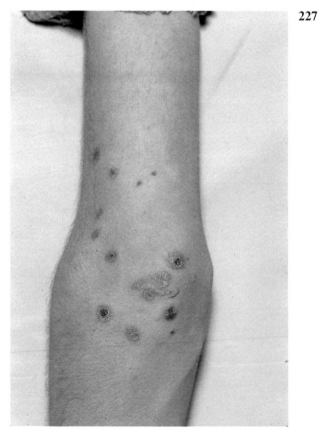

227 Polyarteritis nodosa (PAN) presents with necrotising arteritis in the form of cutaneous papules and/or nodules, usually over the limbs as shown in the antecubital fossa of this 45-year-old woman.

228 Purpura in polyarteritis nodosa. This may not be palpable, and it may affect end arteries as in the digital vessels of this 59-year-old man's toes. This may cause ischaemia and, occasionally, frank gangrene.

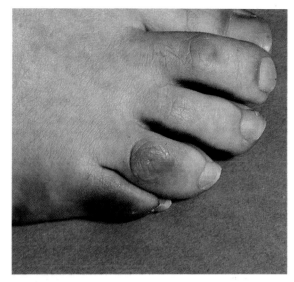

HENOCH-SCHÖNLEIN PURPURA

Children are most commonly affected, following a streptococcal infection or ingestion of drugs, e.g. nonsteroidal anti-inflammatory drugs. A vasculitis associated with cutaneous, gastrointestinal and renal involvement occurs. Malaise, fever, arthralgia, haematuria and abdominal colic may be present. Sero-haemorrhagic effusion into the wall of the gut may cause pain, melaena and intussusception. The platelet count and clotting screen are normal. The condition is usually self limiting, requiring bed rest and analgesia. Severe renal involvement may lead to the nephrotic syndrome.

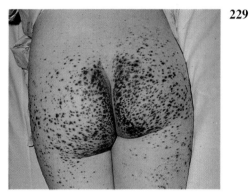

229

229 Henoch-Schönlein purpura (HSP). This occurs on the buttocks and limbs of children and adolescents. In this teenage patient—as often happens—the attack followed a streptococcal upper respiratory tract infection. It resolved within a few weeks.

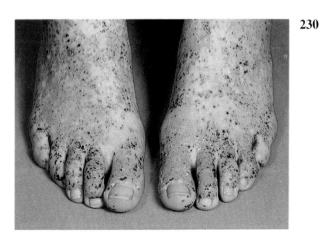

230

230 Purpura in HSP is palpable. This suggests a type III hypersensitivity reaction, resulting in vasculitis. The degree of systemic effect is variable.

POLYMYALGIA RHEUMATICA AND TEMPORAL ARTERITIS

The relationship between polymyalgia rheumatica and temporal or giant cell arteritis is sufficiently close for the two disorders to be regarded as different manifestations of the same process. The former is more common, but arteritis can be found in 50 per cent of patients.

Both conditions occur in the elderly, and their onset may be insidious or abrupt, with malaise, weight loss and low grade fever. The myalgia involves tenderness, stiffness and aching of proximal muscles. Synovitis is common, not only in the shoulders and hips, but also in the knees, where it may be clinically apparent.

Temporal arteritis is an important cause of headache in the elderly; early diagnosis and treatment is essential to remove the risk of blindness from involvement of the posterior ciliary arteries and the central retinal artery branches. Blindness in one or both eyes occurs in 30 per cent of untreated patients. The other cerebral and coronary vessels are rarely affected.

Investigations in both conditions may reveal a normochromic anaemia, a high erythrocyte sedimentation rate (ESR) and raised acute phase proteins, but leucocytosis is absent. Temporal artery biopsy will reveal a necrotizing patchy arteritis, with large mononuclear cell infiltration and giant cells.

Treatment of both conditions involves systemic corticosteroids; their early administration in temporal arteritis may prevent blindness. Temporal arteritis often occurs in isolation, but polymyalgia rheumatica may be a manifestation of occult malignancy, early rheumatoid arthritis or a chronic infection such as bacterial endocarditis.

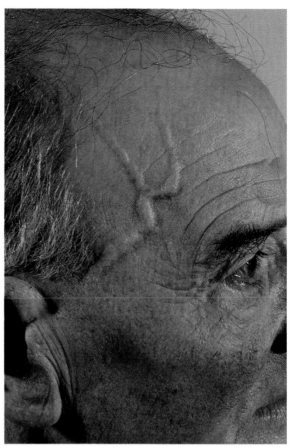

231 Temporal arteritis. This is also known as giant cell arteritis or cranial arteritis. A 74-year-old man developed severe headache, with burning and tenderness over his scalp. His right temporal arteries were very prominent and tender. Biopsy confirmed the diagnosis of giant cell arteritis and he was treated immediately with systemic steroids.

RHEUMATOID ARTHRITIS

This is a common condition, affecting all races and females more commonly than males. It is a multisystem disorder, which may include arteritis, peripheral neuropathy lung and pleural involvement (181 and 182), pericarditis, eye involvement (Chapter 5) and normochromic normocytic ànaemia. Because of its chronicity, the disease may ultimately be complicated by amyloidosis.

Rheumatoid factor is found in most patients, especially when subcutaneous nodules are present. Rheumatoid factor is an antiglobulin, most commonly an IgM which reacts with human IgG. It is also found in up to 30 per cent of patients with SLE, PAN, scleroderma and dermatomyositis.

Treatment of rheumatoid arthritis may include bed rest, local therapy, systemic drug therapy with nonsteroidal anti-inflammatory drugs, and more potent but hazardous agents such as gold, penicillamine, chloroquine and corticosteroids if necessary.

232 Rheumatoid arthritis affecting the meta-carpophalangeal and proximal interphalangeal joints of the hands. There is also wasting of the small muscles of the hand and ulnar deviation due to subluxation.

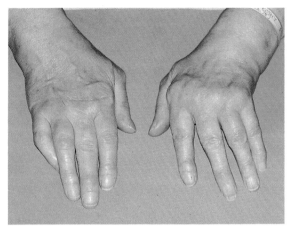

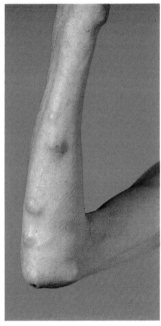

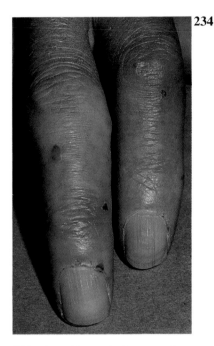

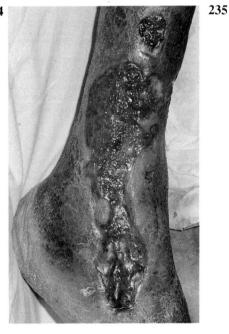

233 Subcutaneous nodules. These are present in 25 per cent of sero-positive rheumatoid arthritis patients (i.e. those in whom rheumatoid factor is present). Nodules are often linked with severe destructive disease.

234 Arteritic lesions characteristically produce nail fold infarcts and splinter necrosis in the digital pulp. Raynaud's phenomenon is also common.

235 Leg ulceration in rheumatoid arthritis. This may result from necrotizing arteritis affecting larger vessels with secondary skin ischaemia. As here, the ulcers are frequently extensive, and a common site is on the lateral aspect of the tibia.

Table 42.   Investigation in autoimmune diseases

	Rheumatoid factor	ANF	LE Cells	DNA antibodies >30%	Serum complement
Systemic lupus erythematosus	20-40%	100%	70-80%	80-100%	N or ↓
Sjögren's syndrome	75-100%	40-70%	10-20%	10-70%	N
Rheumatoid arthritis	70-80%	10-20%	5-10%	0-10%	N+
Scleroderma	4-10%	40-60%*	0-5%	0-10%	N
Polyarteritis nodosa	0-5%	0-5%	0-5%	0-5%	N
Dermatomyositis	0-5%	10-20%	0-5%	0-5%	N

+ Serum complement may be raised during acute inflammation as an 'acute phase' reactant.
* Speckled or nucleolar pattern frequent.

Table 43.   Classification of arteritis

Primary

Polyarteritis nodosa
Granulomatous arteritis (including Wegener's)
Allergic and cutaneous vasculitis
Takaysu's arteritis
Giant cell arteritis

Secondary

Systemic lupus erythematosus
Rheumatoid arthritis
Scleroderma
Childhood dermatomyositis

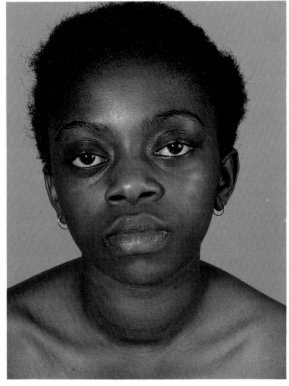

236   Hashimoto's disease commonly presents in women with a firm nodular goitre. Lymphocyte infiltration of the gland, and autoantibodies to thyroglobulin and to thyroid microsomes are to be expected. This teenage patient is rather unusual—the disease most commonly affects middle-aged women.

HASHIMOTO'S DISEASE (autoimmune thyroiditis)

This condition affects mainly middle-aged women and is associated with various autoantibodies. It may present early with transient thyrotoxicosis, or later with hypothyroidism. Other autoimmune disorders may be associated with this disease.

The goitre must be distinguished from other types of non-toxic goitre and from carcinoma of the thyroid. Treatment of hypothyroidism usually requires thyroxine to suppress TSH, cause the gland to diminish in size, and relieve any symptoms of hypothroidism if present.

GRAVES' DISEASE

Patients with Graves' disease are thyrotoxic. They develop a diffuse goitre, exophthalmos, eyelid lag and occasionally pre-tibial myxoedema. Investigation reveals a TSH-like IgG immunoglobulin. Pituitary TSH is suppressed. The presence of 'long acting thyroid stimulator' (LATS) acting on the whole gland and other tissues helps to explain the various clinical features, which are not purely a consequence of elevated levels of thyroxine or tri-iodothyronine. Treatment involves suppressing thyroid overactivity with drugs, radioactive iodine or surgery.

237

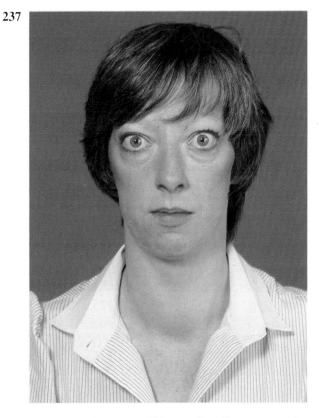

238

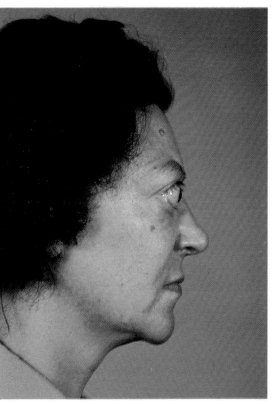

237 Graves' disease. This usually affects women between 20 and 40 years of age. This patient presented classically with a diffuse goitre over which a vascular bruit could be heard.

238 Exophthalmos may occur as a result of mucopolysaccharide infiltration of the orbit or the extraocular muscles which may also cause ophthalmoplegia.

ADDISON'S DISEASE

Atrophy of the adrenal gland in the presence of autoantibodies is now the commonest cause of deficient corticosteroid production. Patients present with weakness, anorexia and gastrointestinal upset. Occasionally they may be hypotensive, hypoglycaemic and hypothermic, with vitiligo and alopecia. If the disease is not treated, coma and death may result.

Investigations reveal hypothalamic (CRF)–pituitary (ACTH)–adrenocortical system failure. The plasma ACTH level indicates directly whether the condition is of primary adrenal origin or the result of an abnormality of the hypothalamic–pituitary system. Treatment is based on glucocorticoid and mineralocorticoid replacement.

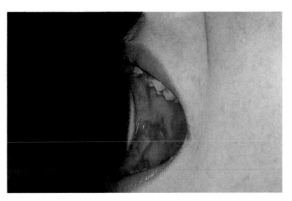

239 Addison's disease with increased ACTH levels causes increased pigmentation, especially of the gums and buccal mucosa.

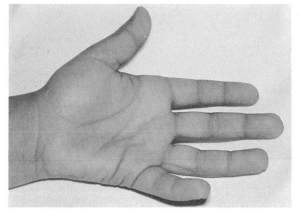

240 Pigmentation in Addison's disease also occurs in skin creases and scars.

PERNICIOUS ANAEMIA

This is primarily a disease of the gastric mucosa in elderly patients. The stomach fails to produce hydrochloric acid, pepsin and intrinsic factor. Gastric cytoplasmic antibodies are present in 80 per cent of patients. Vitamin B_{12} is not absorbed in the absence of gastric intrinsic factor. As a result, patients may develop prematurely grey hair, a macrocytic anaemia, multilobular granulocytes and thrombocytopenia. Rarely subacute degeneration of the cord may occur. Serum B_{12} levels and the Schilling test confirm the diagnosis. Treatment involves B_{12} replacement.

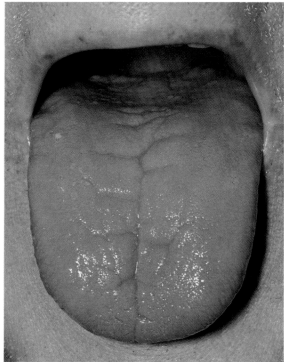

241 Pernicious anaemia. This may present with recurrent soreness of the tongue which is found to be smooth on examination.

MYASTHENIA GRAVIS

This condition is characterised by abnormal fatigue of striated muscle with recovery after rest. There is a reduction in the number of functioning post-synaptic acetylcholine receptors and a high titre of antibodies to these receptors. Thymoma is associated in 15 per cent of cases. Treatment includes neostigmine or pyridostigmine. Thymectomy in some cases appears to increase the chance of remission. An alternate day regime of steroids is of proven value and immunotherapy may be useful. In intractable cases, plasmapheresis has been used.

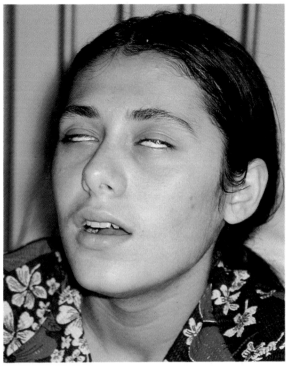

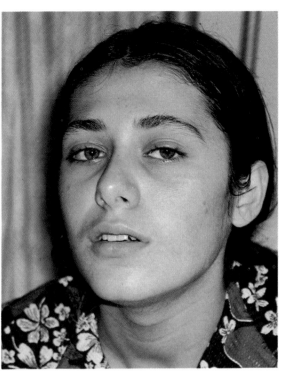

242 Myasthenia gravis can be diagnosed with edrophonium, which temporarily corrects the ptosis resulting from muscle weakness. This picture shows the patient in the fatigued state.

243 Ptosis relieved immediately after an injection of edrophonium 10 mg i.v.

10 IMMUNODEFICIENCY

Immunodeficiency diseases are uncommon but subtle defects in humoral and cellular immunity are being recognised increasingly frequently. The current epidemic of the acquired immune deficiency syndrome (AIDS) has led to a sudden expansion of interest in the nature and causes of immunodeficiency.

A failure of any part of the immune system predisposes an individual to infection, and when children are affected they often also develop type I allergies and rare neoplasms. In adult life a depressed immune response is usually secondary (see Table 44). In most cases, a mild degree of immunodeficiency is of minor relevance to the clinical picture, but it may 'mask' the underlying disease.

Table 44. Causes of secondary inmunosupression in adults

Malnutrition[*]

Infection e.g. rubella[*], Epstein Barr virus, human immunodeficiency virus (HIV)[*]

Drugs e.g. cytotoxics, steroids, antibiotics, phenytoin

Major surgery including splenectomy

Renal failure[*]

Protein losing states

Leukaemia

Lymphomia[*]

The decline accompanying old age

[*] Particularly important causes.

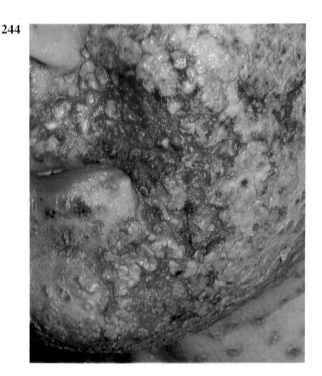

244 Impetiginized herpes simplex infection. This can be severe in patients with diminished cell-mediated immunity and in atopic eczema, as shown here in a 15-year-old girl.

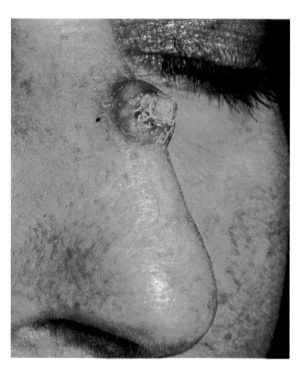

245 Keratoacanthoma may develop in immunosuppressed patients such as this 30-year-old woman who has a renal transplant and is receiving oral cyclosporin A. The histology may sometimes be that of squamous cell carcinoma.

LYMPHORETICULAR MALIGNANCIES

The frequency of opportunistic infections in patients with disseminated malignancy suggests an underlying immune defect, but it is often difficult to distinguish the immunosuppressive effects of the disease from those of the treatment.

Chronic lymphatic leukaemia is commonly complicated by hypogammoglobulinaemia. The serum IgM is usually the first to fall, but panhypogammaglobulinaemia is not uncommon. In a few cases, replacement immunoglobulins provide partial protection.

Acute leukaemia and non-Hodgkin's lymphoma may be associated with both humoral and cell-mediated immunity. The latter is also impaired in Hodgkin's disease. However, the severity of the primary condition usually over-rides the clinical importance of such defects.

Myeloma is often associated with immunoparesis which helps to distinguish it from benign paraproteinaemia. IgM is often the first class to be affected. Immunoglobulin replacement therapy may be helpful, but elimination of the malignant clones leads to a return in immunocompetence.

ACQUIRED IMMUNE DEFICIENCY SYNDROME (AIDS)

This new epidemic form of secondary immunodeficiency usually manifests itself as an opportunistic infection with organisms such as *Pneumocystis carinii*, *Toxoplasma* or *Cytomegalovirus*. In addition, affected patients may have chronic lymphadenopathy, T helper cell lymphopenia and Kaposi's sarcoma. It is caused by the Human Immunodeficiency Virus (HIV) previously known as the Human T-lymphotropic virus type III (HTLV III) or the lymphadenopathy associated virus (LAV). This is a retrovirus, transmitted in semen, saliva and blood, which initially affected mainly homosexual men, drug abusers and haemophiliacs, although it is also transmitted heterosexually. This route is the major cause of the many cases of AIDS in Africa, and is of increasing concern in the rest of the world.

The HIV is cytopathic to some of the mature T helper lymphocytes entering via the interleukin 2 receptor and in which it replicates, and it may cause profound immune deficiency over a period of months or years. A screening test for HIV antibody is available, but it does not predict which patients will develop the lethal condition. Fully established AIDS is fatal and to date there is no known effective treatment.

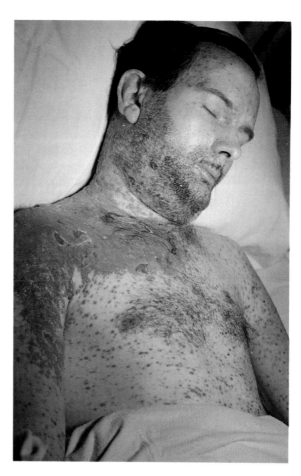

246 Widespread herpes zoster infection in a 38-year-old man developed as a severe complication of Hodgkin's disease.

247

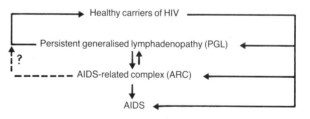

247 The clinical manifestations of HIV infection. Initial infection with HIV commonly causes an influenza or glandular fever-like illness. The following asymptomatic period may last for years, and may, indeed, develop no further, but later there may be persistent weight loss, intermittent fever, chronic diarrhoea, generalised lymphadenopathy, progressive encephalopathy and complex opportunistic infections. Some of those infected with the virus may not go on to develop AIDS, and the factors involved in this progression are not fully understood.

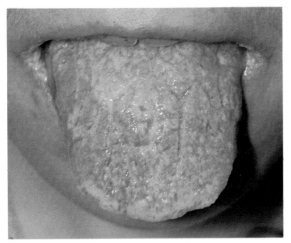

248 Chronic buccal candidiasis. In young men especially, this should alert clinicians to the possible diagnosis of HIV disease.

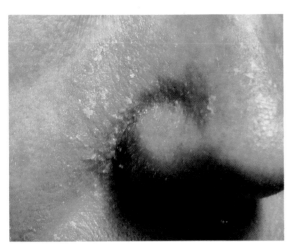

249 'Seborrhoeic dermatitis'. This is common in adults, but it is particularly likely to develop with HIV infection.

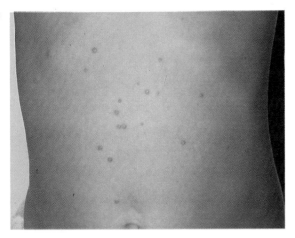

250 Molluscum contagiosum infection. This appears as clusters of pearly papules, which become umbilicated as they grow. It can present in patients infected with HIV, and like a number of other 'minor' infections, it seems to be commoner in 'healthy' carriers than in the normal population.

251

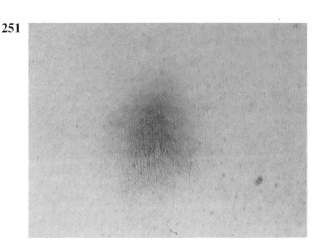

251, 252, 253 Kaposi's sarcoma (multiple idiopathic haemorrhagic sarcoma). This is a rare tumour which presents with slowly enlarging purple or brownish nodules. They may be initially asymptomatic, but Kaposi's sarcoma is one of the major criteria in the diagnosis of full-blown AIDS, and its development is usually associated with symptomatic opportunistic infections.

253

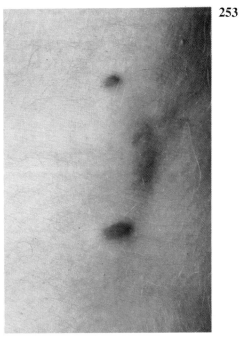

252

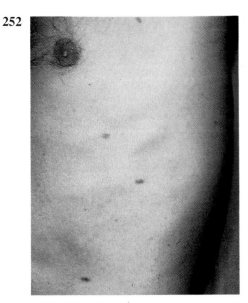

255

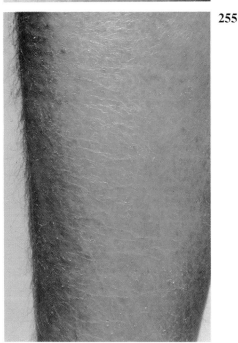

254

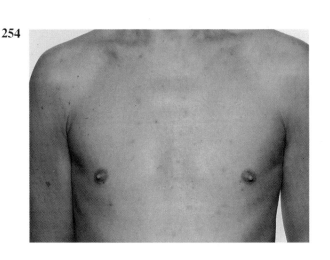

254 Folliculitis and/or papular eczema has recently been recognised as a cutaneous eruption which is commoner in HIV carriers than in the general population.

255 Dry skin (xeroderma) is common, and often non-specific. If acquired by a patient in a high risk group, it may be a pointer to possible infection with HIV.

Table 45. Cutaneous manifestations which may be associated with HIV infection*

- Seborrhoeic dermatitis
- Folliculitis
- Acne vulgaris
- Xeroderma
- Fungal infections
- Herpes simplex
- Impetigo
- Drug eruptions
- Urticaria
- Vasculitis
- Alopecia
- Severe psoriasis
- Granuloma annulare
- Yellow nail syndrome

*Note that most of these conditions are common and benign in the absence of HIV infection.

Table 46. Secondary infections associated with HIV infection

- Oral candidiasis, especially in men
- 'Seborrhoeic dermatitis'
- Folliculitis and/or papular eczema
- Herpes zoster
- Herpes simplex, especially anal infection
- Molluscum contagiosum
- Impetigo contagiosa
- Cellulitis

256

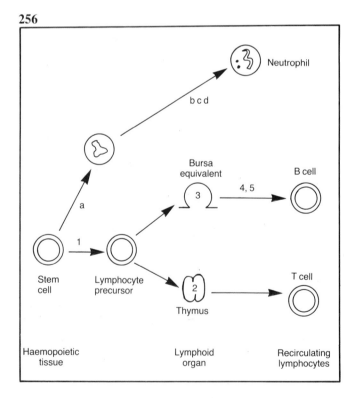

256 Primary immune deficiencies and their principal sites of disorder.

Key

1 Severe combined immunodeficiency
2 Thymic aplasia (Di George's syndrome)
3 X-linked hypogammaglobulinaemia (Bruton's disease)
4 Non-familial hypogammaglobulinaemia
5 Selective immunoglobulin deficiency
Others
    Wiskott-Aldrich syndrome
    Purine nucleoside phosphorylase deficiency
    Adenosine deaminase deficiency

Neutrophil defects
a Primary chronic neutropenia
b Chediak-Higashi syndrome
c Chronic granulomatous disease
d Glucose-6-phosphate dehydrogenase deficiency

Complement deficiencies
C_2 complement component
C_3 complement component

SEVERE COMBINED IMMUNODEFICIENCY

This condition is characterised by a severe defect in humoral and cell-mediated immunity leading to potentially lethal fungal, bacterial and protozoal infections. *Pneumocystis carinii* pneumonia often causes death.

The condition presents from birth as failure to thrive with malabsorption, gut infections and diarrhoea. Clinically the thymus and the tonsils are absent, and there is severe leucopenia. Investigation may reveal adenosine deaminase deficiency in red blood cells and deoxyadenosine in the urine. Low levels of circulating T cells are diagnostic. **Death usually occurs by the age of two.**

The treatment of choice is bone marrow transplantation. Thymus graft and thymic hormone injections have been reported as beneficial.

THYMIC APLASIA (Di George's Syndrome)

Abnormal embryogenesis of the third and fourth pharangeal pouches results in failure of development of the thymus, parathyroids and parts of the cardiovascular system. Neonatal tetany is the first symptom, usually followed by candidiasis and other infections. In a few patients thymus grafts have reversed the immunological defect. Recent reports have suggested benefit from thymic hormone injection therapy.

PARTIAL T CELL DEFECTS

Ataxia telangiectasia. This is an autosomal recessive condition, probably caused by the inability to repair DNA damaged by ionising radiation. Thymus hypoplasia is present with atrophy of Purkinje cells and cerebellar nuclei. Patients can develop lymphomas and half have selective IgA and IgG subclass deficiency, therefore suffering from recurrent infections.

Wiskott-Aldrich syndrome. This is an X-linked recessive disorder and is due to an abnormality in the plasma membrane of platelets and lymphocytes. Patients are prone to infection but also have thrombocytopenia, raised IgE and inability to make IgM to polysaccharide antigen. Affected children are often atopic, suffer from eczema and may die as teenagers from infection, B cell lymphoma and/or cerebral haemorrhage. The treatment of choice is bone marrow transplantation.

X-LINKED HYPOGAMMAGOLBULINAEMIA (Bruton's disease)

Male infants are affected with recurrent viral and bacterial infections from the age of 6 months onwards, having been protected to that time by passively transferred maternal antibody. Eczema is common. All serum immunoglobulins are undetectable, and there are no circulating B cells. Treatment with appropriate antibiotics is essential, with weekly intramuscular immunoglobulin injections. Regular infusions of fresh frozen plasma may be helpful.

NON-FAMILIAL HYPOGAMMAGLOBULIN-AEMIA

This category embraces a heterogeneous group of disorders presenting in childhood or adult life. The clinical features depend on the severity of the antibody deficiency. Despite normal circulating B and T cells, levels of immunoglobulin G, A or M may be low. These can also be selective, and IgA deficiency predisposes the patient to upper respiratory tract infections and diarrhoea from small bowel bacterial overgrowth. Interestingly, selective IgA deficiency is commoner in atopic patients, perhaps suggesting an association between atopy and increased intestinal permeability to ingested antigens. If necessary, treatment is with regular immunoglobulin replacement.

NEUTROPHIL DEFECTS

Primary chronic neutropenia. This is a collection of inherited conditions with variable severity, affecting mainly children. The commonest symptoms are recurrent infections. Prophylactic antibiotics and systemic corticosteroids are beneficial in severe cases.

Chediak-Higashi syndrome. An autosomal recessive disease, in which patients develop respiratory tract and pyogenic skin infections, associated with hepatosplenomegaly and lymphadenopathy. Neutrophil bactericidal and chemotactic activity is impaired. Leucocytes characteristically contain large lysosomal granules. Many patients may develop a lethal lymphoma-like disease before puberty. In a few, Vitamin C may help, but the treatment of choice is bone marrow transplantation.

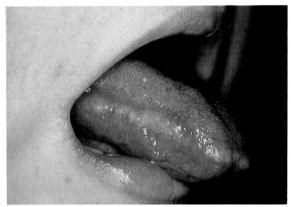

257 Buccal candidiasis with associated oedema of the tongue. This is a common finding in immunosuppressed patients, as in this five-year-old boy with thymic aplasia (Di George's syndrome).

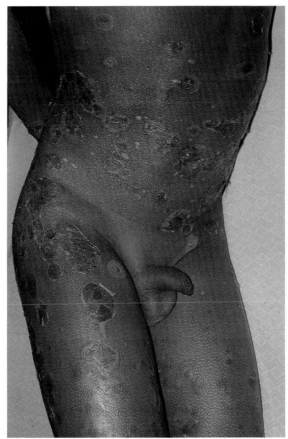

258 Impetigo contagiosa. This is a spreading staphylococcal or streptococcal epidermal infection. It can become widespread, particularly in X-linked hypogammaglobulinaemia (Bruton's disease).

Chronic granulomatous disease. An inherited disorder due to a failure of neutrophils to kill catalase positive bacteria such as *Staphylococcus aureus*. There is a wide spectrum of clinical severity. Patients develop abscesses and salmonellosis of the gut. Prophylactic antibiotics may help, but bone marrow transplantation should be considered.

COMPLEMENT DEFICIENCY
Patients suffer severe life-threatening infections requiring prompt antibiotic therapy. In C_2 deficiency there is an increased incidence of systemic lupus erythematosus.

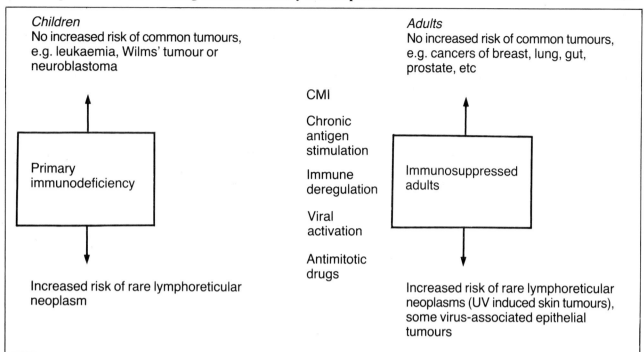

Children
No increased risk of common tumours,
e.g. leukaemia, Wilms' tumour or
neuroblastoma

Primary
immunodeficiency

Increased risk of rare lymphoreticular
neoplasm

CMI

Chronic
antigen
stimulation

Immune
deregulation

Viral
activation

Antimitotic
drugs

Adults
No increased risk of common tumours,
e.g. cancers of breast, lung, gut,
prostate, etc

Immunosuppressed
adults

Increased risk of rare lymphoreticular
neoplasms (UV induced skin tumours),
some virus-associated epithelial
tumours

FURTHER READING

Bull, T. R., *A Colour Atlas of ENT Diagnosis,* Wolfe Medical Publications, London, 1987.

Cormane, R. M. and Ashgar, *Immunology and Skin Disease,* Edward Arnold, London, 1981.

Brostoff, J., and Challacombe, S. J., *Food Allergy and Intolerance,* Bailliere Tindall, London, 1987.

Dahl, M. V., *Clinical Immunodermatology,* Year Book Publishers, Inc., Chicago, Illinois.

Fitzpatrick, T. B., Eisen, A. Z., Wolf, K., Freedberg, I. M., and Austen, K. F., *Dermatology in General Medicine,* (2nd ed), McGraw Hill, Maindenhead, Berks.

James, D. G., and Studdy, P. R., *A Colour Atlas of Respiratory Diseases,* Wolfe Medical Publications, London, 1981.

Lessof, M. H. (Editor), *Allergy: Immunology and Clinical Aspects,* John Wiley & Sons, Chichester, Sussex, 1984.

Lessof, M. H., Lee, T. H. and Kemeny, D. M., (Editors) *Allergy: An International Textbook*, John Wiley & Sons, Chichester, Sussex, 1987.

Lichtenstein, L. M., and Fauci, A. J., *Current Therapy in Allergy, Immunology and Rheumatology,* Decker, 1985.

Miller, D., Weber, J., and Green, J., *The management of AIDS Patients,* Mcmillian, Basingstoke, Hants, 1986.

Mygind, N., *Essential Allergy—An Illustrated Text for Students and Specialists*, Blackwell Scientific, Oxford, 1986.

Roitt, I., Brostoff, J., and Male, D., *Immunology,* Chruchill Livingstone, Edinburgh and Gower Medical Publishing, London, 1985.

Rook, A., Wilkinson, D. S., Ebling, F. J. G., Champion, R. M., and Burton, J. L., *Textbook of Dermatology*, (4th Ed) Blackwell Scientific Publications, Oxford.

Royal College of Physicians and the British Nutrition Foundation, (joint report) 'Food intolerance and Food Aversion', *J. Roy. Coll. Phy.* 1984, **18**, 83-123.

Workman, E., Hunter, J., and Jones, V. A., *The Allergy Diet — How to Overcome Your Food Intolerance*, Martin Dunitz, London, 1984.

INDEX

Figures refer to page numbers

Pseudo-allergic reactions, 8
Purine nucleoside phosphorylase deficiency, 116